The New Drug Reimbursement Game

Brita A.K. Pekarsky

The New Drug Reimbursement Game

A Regulator's Guide to Playing and Winning

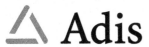 Adis

Brita A.K. Pekarsky
University of South Australia
Adelaide
Australia

ISBN 978-3-319-34920-6   ISBN 978-3-319-08903-4 (eBook)
DOI 10.1007/978-3-319-08903-4
Springer Cham Heidelberg New York Dordrecht London

Printed on acid-free paper

Springer is part of Springer Science+Business Media (www.springer.com)

Foreword

The sustainability of publicly funded health care systems is continually under threat allegedly because of the ageing of the population, new technologies and expectations of the public. Yet none of these factors provide prima facie evidence of increases in the need for care among the population. Demographic change is the result of improvements in average levels of health within age groups; technological change is aimed at improving technical efficiency (producing more from the same, or less) while individuals do not enjoy consuming health care (more is not better) but undergo the often uncomfortable, sometimes painful and occasional lethal processes based on the provider's advice about the expected outcomes. What then explains this constant threat to what are arguably the most popular public policy developments in countries who benefit from universal publicly funded health care? Is there something fundamental in the institutional structure of publicly funded health care systems that cause ever increasing cost escalation together with pressures for policy responses to accommodate these cost escalation by either reducing the number of people covered and/or the range of service covered (privatisation of funding by any other name).

Over 20 years ago, together with my colleague Amiram Gafni, I published a paper that showed the underlying problem was a fundamental flaw in the methods for evaluating the efficiency of new technologies in health care—methods that relied on highly theoretical assumptions and exclusion of consideration of the economic concept of opportunity cost. Despite many attempts to discredit our arguments (or, in some cases, discredit our characters), we continued to observe the costs of health care programmes increase rapidly even though methods that were intended to identify only technologies that improved technical efficiency were being adopted as mandatory elements for inclusion in new programme proposals.

About 10 years ago we recognised that the methods 'pushers' (those responsible for the national, regional and local health authorities becoming 'addicted' to increased spending) were often involved either directly or indirectly with interests (e.g., the pharmaceutical sector) who stood to gain from such cost escalation—a perfect example of Bob Evans' health care income-expenditure identity.

Somehow, somewhere, sometime, somebody needed to generate the toolkit for public agencies to protect them from the poor economic advice on which economic evaluation guidelines are based. That is where Brita Pekarsky's 'The new drug reimbursement game: a regulator's guide to playing and winning' comes in. Based on Brita's Ph.D. thesis at the University of Adelaide, it develops the methodology for decision makers to negate the impact of the invalid assumptions of the 'pushers' and identify the social value of new technologies within the real world in which regulators operate. I recommend a careful reading of the book by anyone involved with or interested in the area of health care regulation and economic appraisal of health care technologies. It bridges the divide between the economic concept of technical efficiency and the practical challenges of finding value for money in health care and offers the prospect of adopting planning and evaluation methods that support and contribute towards sustainability of our publicly funded health care systems.

Hamilton, ON, Canada   Steve Birch
2013

Acknowledgements

This book is based on my Ph.D. thesis, which was completed while I held a Divisional Scholarship awarded by the University of Adelaide. The generous advice and guidance provided by my Ph.D. supervisors—Professor Jon Karnon, Dr. Virgine Masson and Professor Simon Eckermann—was invaluable.

From 1997 to 2013 I was a member of the Economic Subcommittee of the Australian Pharmaceutical Benefits Advisory Committee. My understanding of the pharmaceutical regulation process is largely attributable to Mr. Andrew Mitchell and Professor Lloyd Samson.

Mr. Sunjay Pekarsky-Norman assisted me in the preparation of this manuscript: preparing figures, testing styles, discussing grammar and editing.

Abbreviations

AUSFTA	Australia–U.S. Free Trade Agreement
aICER	Average incremental cost-effectiveness ratio
CBA	Cost benefit analysis
CEA	Cost-effectiveness analysis
CEA_i	Cost-effectiveness analysis applied in conjunction with a threshold of i
CSIRO	Commonwealth Scientific and Industrial Research Organization
CVI	Clinical value of innovation
DTM	Decision theoretic model
EBM	Evidence-based medicine
EVCI	Economic value of clinical innovation
FCUSS	Finance Committee of the US Senate
FDA	Food and Drug Administration
FPP	Firm's preferred price (per effect of a new drug)
FTA	Free trade agreement
GDP	Gross domestic product
GTM	Game theoretic model
HTA/CEA	Health technology assessment/cost-effectiveness analysis
ICER	Incremental cost-effectiveness ratio
IMER	Incremental manufacturing cost-effectiveness ratio
IMS Health	Not an abbreviation but the name of a pharmaceutical data company
IPER	Incremental price-effectiveness ratio
ITA	International Trade Administration (US Government)
maxWTP	maximum Willingness To Pay
NB	Net benefit
NICE	National Institute for Health and Clinical Excellence
NME	New molecular entity
npvPH	Net present value of the population's health
npvSW	Net present value social welfare
OECD	Organisation for Economic Cooperation and Development

PBAC	Pharmaceutical Benefits Advisory Committee
PBMA	Programme budgeting marginal analysis
PBS	Pharmaceutical Benefits Scheme
PEA	Price-effectiveness analysis
PEND	Political economy of new drugs
Pharma	The pharmaceutical industry
PhRMA	Pharmaceutical Researcher and Manufacturers of America
PPP	Purchaser's preferred price
QALY	Quality adjusted life year
R&D	Research and development
RCT	Randomised controlled trial
RSA	Risk-sharing agreement
WHO	World Health Organisation

Contents

Chapter 1
Introduction

Abstract New drug reimbursement is a high stakes game and price is the mechanism whereby the new drug's innovative surplus is apportioned between consumers and producers. Some countries use the results of cost-effectiveness analyses to inform the pricing decision. These countries express the result of a cost-effectiveness analysis as a price per effect and compare it to a decision threshold; a price above which the regulator will consider rejecting the new drug. Typically, if a decision threshold is lower that the firm's preferred price (FPP) and there is a possibility of rejection, a firm will mount an evidence based case as to why the final drug price should not be below the threshold. There is a plethora of texts and guidelines available to regulators and health economic analysts on the methods of cost-effectiveness analyses of new drugs and the choice of decision thresholds. There are few, if any, formal texts available to guide regulators as to the optimal response to the claim that prices below the FPP are not in the population's best interest because the benefits of cost saving today are offset by the loss of *future* health due to less innovation. This chapter introduces four rules and four tools which, if applied by regulators, will maximise the present value of the population's health. A key theme is introduced: a strategy used by firms in the new drug reimbursement game is the threat that lower prices are not in the interest of the population.

1.1 The Regulator's Challenge

At a time when evidence-based medicine increasingly dominates decision-making and health budgets are tightened, how should institutions respond to the following ostensibly evidence-based claim?

- Lowering the price of a new drug below the firm's preferred price will lead to *suboptimal* investments in research and development (R&D) and lower health for the population than otherwise possible.

For institutions that use economic evaluation and decision thresholds to guide decisions about new drugs, this problem comes down to the following question:

© Springer International Publishing Switzerland 2015
B.A.K. Pekarsky, *The New Drug Reimbursement Game*,
DOI 10.1007/978-3-319-08903-4_1

- What should the new drug decision threshold be, given the dynamic efficiency implications of the relationship between new drug price and the health benefits of future drugs?

Unsurprisingly, the debate surrounding this question is highly charged. "New drug price"[1] impacts both health and profits. Hence, this book starts with the economic expression of the debate; the political economy of new drugs. The active participants of this political economy include academics, industry, regulators, consumers and global organisations such as the World Health Organization (WHO) and the Organisation for Economic Cooperation and Development (OECD).

The research question addressed in this book has its origins in four observations by Comanor (1986). First, he found that the political economy of the pharmaceutical industry has shaped economists' research agenda since the Kefauver Committee of 1959.[2] He also noted that changes in the research agenda were driven by changes in the political debate. Second, Comanor found that the one research question common to the disparate literature on the subject was an estimate of the ratio of investment in R&D to the social return on this investment. However, he also found there was no methodologically-sound estimate of this ratio at the time of his publication (1986). Third, he observed that the antagonistic nature of the political debate is reflected in two distinct positions held by economists: (1) unregulated monopoly power by firms is essential to ensure there is sufficient innovation for the population; and (2) regulation is necessary to ensure that social welfare gains from pharmaceuticals are maximised. Finally, he also noted that the then (1986) current political economy, and hence research agenda, excluded one possible outcome of more competition (lower prices) today, namely, improved social welfare tomorrow. Hence, the trade-off that characterises the political economy might not exist under all regulatory structures; it could be possible to have more competition as well as more innovation and better health tomorrow.

Inspired by these observations, I started this research by reframing the political economy in a way that will allow the economic research to find a solution to the choice of a decision threshold that maximises population health and also takes into

---

[1] Throughout this book I use the term "new drug price" in the context of new drug prices generally. If a specific price is referred to I use the term "the price of the new drug" or "the new drug's price". See "Glossary of Phrases".

[2] Kefauver was a US Congressman then Senator from 1939 to his death in 1963. He chaired a number of significant US Senate Committees, including a 1950 committee on organised crime. The Kefauver Committee of 1959 was motivated by the "excess profits" of the US pharmaceutical industry. It was seen as an antitrust (market power) Committee rather than a drug safety and quality regulation Committee. His work on this Committee resulted in the Kefauver-Harris Drug Act of 1962. This committee explored the nature and consequences of market power and rent seeking in the pharmaceutical industry. Amongst other things, it challenged the pharmaceutical industry's payments to the American Medical Association in terms of the implications this would have for objective scientific reporting of new drugs. For further information, a good place for an economist to start is Comanor (1966).

account the relationship between price and innovation. This alternative to the conventional political economy is framed from the perspective of an institution that is required to select and then enforce a decision threshold price that maximises the net present value of the population's health (npvPH). It starts with the following characterisation of the debate.

> Higher prices today mean increased economic rent for the pharmaceutical industry (Pharma) otherwise firms would not lobby for them. It is in Pharma's interest to protect and seek these economic rents. Whether higher prices and more R&D today increase future health remains an empirical question. If higher prices also mean a higher *net* present value of the population's health, then it is in the institution's interest to increase prices. Given the institution's objectives, the most effective strategy Pharma can use to protect these rents is "the Threat": lowering prices is against the interest of health funders because it will reduce a population's future health.

The regulator's challenge is to answer the following question:

- "How should rational institutions respond to the Threat?"

(A rational response is one that is consistent with a given institution's stated objective function, whatever this may be.)

This introduction places this research question in the context of current evidence and research, by addressing the following three questions.

- Is it plausible that the Threat exists and that it influences the price of new drugs?
- Is there rigorous empirical evidence that suggests that lower drug prices will result in reduced future health?
- Are economists in agreement as to the value of a decision threshold for new drugs that accommodates characteristics of the health budget such as allocative and technical inefficiency?

Then the method used in this book to explore the research question is summarised and the structure of the book is outlined.

1.2 Is It Plausible That the Threat Exists and That it Influences the Price of New Drugs?

1.2.1 What Is a Threat?

The claim by the pharmaceutical industry that lower prices today will make the population worse off is appropriately characterised as a threat. In game theory, a threat is simply a claim by one player about his or her future behaviour, conditional on the decisions made by another player, today.[3] This claim could be credible or, quite simply, a lie. The important point is that a threat is telling a player to consider the likely response by another player when making a decision. In the case of the price of new drugs, the pharmaceutical industry uses a range of threats to provide an incentive for an institution not to lower prices in order to make savings today. For example, a firm could state: "If your country lowers prices, we will not invest in innovation and there will be no more new drugs in the future". In game theory the issue is how the institution should respond to this threat, given what is known about the firm and its motives.

The particular threat that is the subject of this book (the Threat) is likely to be operating throughout the OECD, including the US. Of particular interest in this research is the influence that the Threat has in countries that: (1) have universal health care; (2) have budget constraints; (3) have a fund holder with the broad objective of maximising a population's health and welfare[4]; (4) inform drug reimbursement decisions with health technology assessment/cost-effectiveness analysis (HTA/CEA)[5]; and (5) use an explicit or implicit decision threshold price in a new drug adoption decision where this threshold is expressed as an average incremental cost per unit incremental effect [incremental cost-effectiveness ratio, (ICER)].

It is possible that the Threat is present (either explicitly or implicitly) each time an institution decides whether to reimburse a drug that has a high ICER compared with the institution's decision threshold. If this does occur in the private domain, it cannot be used as evidence in academic research. However, the Threat does dominate international debate about drug price regulation, and this debate is largely in the public domain. The case of the Australia–US Free Trade Agreement (AUSFTA) negotiations is one such example.

---

[3] See for example, Gibbons (1992), p. 56.

[4] Of course this is a simplistic definition of the objective of a health care system. The main point is that this system does not explicitly value the following as part of the drug reimbursement process: the technology that is used to deliver the health gains. That is, whatever it is that the health system values, it is irrelevant to the Reimburser's decision whether the outcome is obtained using the newest drug or conventional old tech therapies. Specifically, this excludes the possibility that a clinical or institutional decision maker will be prepared to pay for "novelty". The possibility that this is the case is raised in the Conclusion.

[5] Relative to the early adopters (Australia and Canada) some European countries are late adopters of routine use of economic evaluation to inform drug decisions (post 2000), and the US is still to adopt this practice. How early did Australia and Canada start using economic evaluation of pharmaceuticals? From the 1994 first edition of the Canadian Economic Evaluation Guidelines: *"Australia was the first country to develop and implement guidelines for the economic evaluation of pharmaceuticals. Draft guidelines were released in 1990, revised in 1992, and are currently going through the process of second revision. In Canada, the process for developing these guidelines began when the Province of Ontario issued draft guidelines for comment in the Fall of 1991. During 1992 it was determined that it would be useful to develop a set of Canadian guidelines, that each Province could adopt, with or without modifications, as they saw fit"* (Canadian Coordinating Office for Health Technology Assessment 1994).

1.2.2   A Public Domain Expression of This Threat: The Australian–US FTA

In 2004, the negotiations between Australia and the US that resulted in the AUSFTA were almost derailed when the Australian practice of regulating the price of pharmaceuticals was challenged by the US government, which claimed this practice went against the principles of free trade.[6] The US government argued that the Australian practice of using cost-effectiveness analysis (CEA) to inform reimbursement decisions resulted in lower prices in Australia than in the US. Australia was therefore a free-rider on the significant investments made by US consumers into pharmaceutical R&D via higher drug prices. Furthermore, as a consequence of OECD-wide policies, including those of Australia, US consumers had to pay higher prices for the same drugs in order that firms could continue to finance pharmaceutical R&D; R&D that Australians were likely to benefit from in future. The records of the Congress and US Senate Committees are rich with references to this debate, in particular, the 204-page document that is the record of a joint hearing of two subcommittees of the Finance Committee of the US Senate. Consider the opening remarks of this Joint Hearing, made by the Chair of the Health Care Subcommittee:

> I have long thought that the prescription drug price controls employed by foreign countries amount to an unfair trade practice because they block the access of U.S. product to foreign markets, but worse is that the price controls impose unacceptable burdens on the United States as our consumers end up paying the bulk of the cost for research and development, probably up to 60 % more for most prescription drugs compared to the citizens and countries that use price controls. Hon. Jon Kyl, U.S. Senator From Arizona, Chairman, Subcommittee On Health Care (Finance Committee US Senate 2004)

Moreover, the opening remarks from the Chairman of the Subcommittee on International Trade reveal a concern for "the folks in Australia" should they reduce their control on pharmaceutical prices, but that this was a requirement of an AUSFTA on which the US was not prepared to compromise:

> So I think that price setting is sort of, in a way, similar to a tariff that is put on the goods. It has a great impact on what happens here. To deal with these, Congress passed the Trade Act of 2002, which established a primary objective of tightening the regulatory practices that create market distortions and effectively deny U.S. companies global access. As we know, the issue of regulatory practices relating to pharmaceuticals was one of the last items resolved in the recently completed Australian Free Trade Agreement negotiations. It is a sensitive issue for the folks in Australia, and I respect their concerns. But it is an issue that deserved to be on the table, and one that needs to be raised in future negotiations. Hon. Craig Thomas, a U.S. Senator from Wyoming, Chairman, Subcommittee On International Trade (Finance Committee US Senate 2004)

Not only was pharmaceutical price regulation characterised as anti-competitive and analogous to tariffs on imports, it was also argued to reduce incentives for

---

[6] A summary of the issues is contained in Harvey et al. (2004).

innovation and hence the number of new drugs available in future. The US government argued that, as a consequence of widespread price controls, the health of the OECD's population was less than what would otherwise be possible. At around the same time as the AUSFTA was being negotiated, a US government agency, the International Trade Administration (ITA), published a report on the implications for US consumers of the OECD countries' practice of price control for new drugs (ITA 2004). This study found that if all OECD countries (apart from the US) stopped regulating drug prices *and* stopped using monopsonist purchasing power there would be an additional three to four new molecular entities (NMEs) each year, a consequence that would have significant positive value to all OECD consumers.

The ITA study also revealed a view amongst US pharma-economists that the process of using a threshold price above which the drug could no longer be considered value for money was price control under another name, and hence the policy could be classified as a trade restriction.

> Cost-effectiveness reviews, called the "fourth hurdle requirements" by industry, are defined as government consideration of "factors other than safety, efficacy, and quality in approving new drugs for marketing or reimbursement." Although the schemes differ from country to country, the determination that a new medicine is not cost-effective or "medically necessary" can work much like price controls because the analysis can be performed in a way that makes clear that a price reduction will make the drug acceptable. (International Trade Administration 2004 p. 6)

1.2.3   The Threat Exists and It Is Plausible That It Influences Decisions

The Threat exists and was applied during AUSFTA trade negotiations. The Finance Committee of the US Senate, US Pharma and US government economists appeared to be almost unanimous in their public position that the Australian Pharmaceutical Benefits Scheme (PBS) and similar institutions are restricting free trade and that this was at a cost to the future health of, not only US citizens, but all of the world's citizens. A notable exception amongst the US pharma-economic literature is Reinhardt's criticism of the free trade argument and the associated estimates of the benefits to the US and other countries of removing price controls.[7] (Reinhardt 2007) It is plausible that this Threat influenced the result of these negotiations, for example, by requiring that the AUSFTA include an additional annex that

---

[7] A second important exception was the statement by Prof. Gerard Anderson, of John Hopkins. His oral statement and the resultant discussion with the Joint Committee Hearing are both reproduced as Attachment 2. These excerpts capture the drama and intensity of the political economy of new drugs perfectly. And finally, Prof. Alan Sager (2003) from Boston School of Public Health gave a presentation in 2003 (around the same time) which summarises the issues regarding access from the position of the US.

acknowledged the requirement for its pricing processes to recognise and reward pharmaceutical innovation.[8]

1.3   What Is the Evidence Upon Which This Threat Is Founded?

If there were unambiguous evidence that lowering a price below the firm's preferred price (FPP) would make a population worse off in terms of the npvPH, then an institution with the objective of maximising population health would presumably prefer to price at the FPP. However, the question of whether such evidence exists, and its applicability to countries outside the US, is a contentious issue.

US pharma-economists have built a significant body of theoretical and empirical evidence that supports but rarely challenges the case for the FPP as the social welfare—and population health—maximising price.[9] However, this body of evidence is not straightforward to assess. For example, there are a number of ways in which this FPP is defined, including: (1) the price that would occur in an unregulated unilateral monopoly market (International Trade Administration 2004); and (2) the maximum willingness to pay (maxWTP) for a health effect (Vernon et al. 2009). Furthermore, the theoretical and empirical analyses supporting the case for the FPP tend to assume that budgets are unconstrained, and thus the applicability of any results to countries that have fixed health budgets and alternatives other than pharmaceutical R&D to invest in and achieve improved future health is limited (see Chap. 3). Finally, the empirical studies that support the unregulated price often draw on private domain databases that are costly to access, and hence the opportunity to analyse these data with models that specify health budgets as constrained (rather than uncapped) is limited.[10] In summary, the empirical and theoretical evidence is not necessarily strong enough to support the case made by US pharma-economists, the US government and their agencies and Pharma.

.

---

[8] See discussion of this issue in Chap. 4.

[9] Not all US pharma-economists claim that existing evidence provides unambiguous support for the FPP. For example, Reinhardt (2007) and Comanor (1986) have critiqued the methods used in some pharma-economic studies.

[10] See for example (Giaccotto et al. 2005) which accessed a data set from Pharmaceutical Researcher and Manufacturers of America (PhRMA) that is not in the public domain.

1.4   What Are the Current Options for the Decision Threshold?

1.4.1   Existing Options for the Decision Threshold

If institutions wish to formally assess the FPP, then they need to compare in to an alternative. Currently, there is no agreed purchaser's preferred price (PPP) or decision threshold that could be compared with any given FPP in terms of its social welfare and health implications. Health economists have been debating the question of the choice of decision threshold price since 1992, for programme adoption generally (Birch and Gafni 1992, 1993; Johannesson and Weinstein 1993) and for drugs specifically (Drummond 1992). Some institutions have claimed that there are no explicit thresholds, but reviews of their decisions seem to suggest otherwise (Devlin and Parkin 2004; George et al. 2001). Around 2007, there was a shift away from support for the maxWTP, which was the preferred threshold of many health economists since 1993,[11,12] (Culyer et al. 2007; McCabe et al. 2008).

One proposed alternative is a threshold of the average ICER of services displaced to finance the new drug, d (Sendi et al. 2002). This threshold is likely to be sensitive to budgetary impact[13] and minimises the risk that the reimbursement of new drugs results in a net reduction in the population's health. However, what if the threshold is revealed by institutions to be d and firms are strategic and price at this threshold? Then the net effect of ongoing displacement and new drug adoption on the population's health is zero; the new drug's innovation improves the health of a group of patients but there is no net gain in the population's health.

Such a result, pharmaceutical innovation being taken up, but having no net impact on a population's health, could be acceptable in a country that places a value on new technology adoption per se, independent of its impact on a population's health. Such a country could make claims such as: "Our country is the first to have all the latest medical technologies available for use by patients". However, if a county's primary rationale for new technology adoption is to improve the population's health from existing resources, then research that found that new technologies were available rapidly, but that there was no net increase in the

---

[11] This preference for using the maxWTP as a threshold price (or "value for money" as a criterion) for adoption and reimbursement probably continues in many institutions. Since 1992 Birch and Gafni have pointed out that this strategy will not maximise a population's health from a given budget, unless the budget is sufficiently large to accommodate all programs that are value for money or that the budget continues to increase to accommodate these programs and technologies.

[12] The National Institute for Health and Clinical Excellence (2007) provides a summary of the issues.

[13] The budgetary impact is the net additional cost of adopting the new drug. The proposed threshold of d will be a function of budgetary impact if the cost per effect of displaced services changes as the amount of services displaced increases. This is in contrast to the most prominent option for the threshold k, the maximum willingness to pay for a health effect, which is exogenous to the state of the health budget.

population's health, could lead that country to question their decision-making processes.

1.4.2   The Health Shadow Price as the Decision Threshold

The research presented in this book proposes a new PPP: the health shadow price, β_c. To derive β_c, this research draws on a conventional cost benefit analysis (CBA) method of deriving a shadow price for an input (in this case, a new drug) in the presence of market failure, by referencing the shadow price of the output (for which there is a market) (McKean 1972; Mishan and Quah 2007). This method can be summarised as defining the price of the input (without the market price) such that the decision maker is indifferent between adopting the strategy that includes that input and adopting the best alternative strategy, where all inputs have a market price. This conventional method is developed further in this book to accommodate a number of characteristics that economists would expect to find in a health sector, including:

- Suboptimal displacement (the services displaced to finance the additional costs of a new drug are not necessarily the least cost-effective of current services); and
- Allocative and technical inefficiency in the health budget.

The result, β_c, is the ICER of a new drug, above which the population would be better off (i.e. the population's health would be greater) if the institution chose the best alternative strategy, rather than the strategy of reimbursement. Improving the allocative or technical efficiency of the health budget is the alternative strategy considered in this book.

1.5   The Framework for This Research

1.5.1   Price-Effectiveness Analysis

This book develops and then applies a framework, price-effectiveness analysis (PEA) to address the research question. This framework accommodates strategic behaviour by both firms and institutions, in addition to the characteristics of the economic context as captured by β_c. The economic method used in this part of the research is applied game theory, which was selected for two reasons.

First, unlike decision theoretic models (DTMs), game theoretic models (GTMs) can capture the consequence of more than one decision maker in the reimbursement process, for example both the firm and the institution, where these players (decision makers) act strategically. Acting strategically means that players consider the response of the other player when they make a decision such as choosing an offer price of a new drug. For example, a firm (which as a monopolist is a price maker) will consider whether or not an institution will reject a new drug at a particular offer price when it selects its offer price.

Second, a theoretical game, like most theoretical economics, is driven largely by making small changes to existing models, which might have very little relevance to the real world of health and economics. For example, consider a theoretically-derived model that makes the following assumptions about the health sector: (1) no budget constraints; (2) perfect and complete (public) information; (3) no strategic behaviour; (4) no failure in the market for evidence of the cost and effect of unpatented and unpatentable services; and (5) economic efficiency. Conventionally, a piece of theoretical research would involve extending such a model by making small changes; for example, assuming that there is a budget constraint. However, the resultant adapted model would struggle to accommodate the characteristics of the health system that generate the very situations that are the subject of health economic research, in particular those that arise because of the complexity of information in the health sector. In contrast, applied game theory draws its inspiration from the real world, rather than existing models, and the challenge is to generate models that capture vital real world characteristics. Therefore, GTMs rather than DTMs were used, and an applied rather than theoretic approach was used to develop these games.

1.5.2   The Role of the Narrative in the Models and the Research

The use of the narrative to capture the vital characteristics of an economic problem is a distinguishing characteristic of game theory. For example, the narrative of the Prisoner's Dilemma[14] is reasonably well known, even if the application of economic theory to solve this game is not. This book also uses a narrative structure to develop models and concepts that capture an increasing number of the characteristics that influence the political economy of new drugs. This narrative takes the form of a series of problems that a Reimburser in a hypothetical country has when she tries to select and then enforce a PPP. Each of the Chaps. 3–11 starts with the Reimburser being presented with a specific dilemma, which is referred to as: The Reimburser's Problem. The narrative uses three main characters (a Reimburser, a Firm and a Health Economic Adviser) to set up and then explore that Chapter's problem.

The secondary cast members are: "pharma-economists", who research and analyse the economics of the industry, pharmaceutical R&D and drug price; and

---

[14] For a description of both the narrative and the associated economic model of the Prisoner's dilemma, see Gibbons (1992).

"pharmaco-economists", who research and analyse the economics of the molecule, patients and the decision threshold.

There are also two key sectors: "Pharma", the pharmaceutical industry; and "the Institution", which is the broad group of government pharmaceutical decision makers, fund holders and regulators. The Firm is a member of the former sector and the Reimburser of the latter.

The narrative approach allows some of the debates and conversations that are common to drug reimbursement processes around the world—and often in the private domain—to be part of the games' narratives and the Reimburser's problems, without attributing specific actions or claims to any particular firm or regulator. The use of capital letters to start terms such as "Firm" and "Institution" is necessary in the context of the three Games (Chaps. 8–10) as this signifies it is a firm or institution with carefully specified characteristics, such as objective and cost functions and decision rules. The use of firm with a small "f" refers to any firm in the pharmaceutical industry. The use of capitals to refer to the Reimburser and the Health Economic Adviser is a literary (rather than methodological) device.

1.6 Overview of Book: Concepts, Tools, Rules of the Game

This book is intended to be a practical guide for health economists advising institutions on the drug pricing process. It is built on six theoretical concepts.

1. The *political economy*, as expressed via the policy narrative, is reframed to identify additional research questions. This research agenda and the associated models are specified so as not to exclude any of the following outcomes of higher drug prices: an improvement, a reduction or no change in the present value of the population's future health.
2. The *opportunity cost of a strategy* in an institutional setting does not necessarily imply that the decision maker is physically choosing between these two strategies and their corresponding end state alternatives. Instead, it means that the decision maker is valuing all states of the world that could emerge under different allocations of resources. This definition is consistent with that proposed by Buchanan (2008).
3. *Price-effectiveness analysis* is a method of assessing the decision to reimburse a new drug by testing the relationship between the price of the new drug and the population's health.
4. The strategy of *reimbursement* comprises the actions of *adoption* (substituting an existing therapy with an alternative) and *financing* (displacing services or expanding the budget to fund the additional cost of the new drug).
5. The *health shadow price*, β_c, is the incremental cost per incremental health effect gained by the target patients as a consequence of the strategy of reimbursing (adopting and financing) the new drug with clinical innovation ΔE and additional financial cost ΔC. At this point, the funder is indifferent between the

strategy of reimbursement and the best alternative strategy (optimal adoption and displacement) available to the funder also using the resources ΔC. The health shadow price is conditional on a given economic context (c) which is defined by existing prices, inefficiency and budget expenditure required.

6. The *economic value of clinical innovation*, $\text{EVCI} = \beta_c \, \Delta E$ is the gross clinical benefit of the new drug compared to placebo, constrained twice: by the clinical opportunity cost (the best alternative therapy to the new drug) to obtain ΔE and the economic opportunity cost (the best alternative use of resources ΔC) to obtain $\beta_c \, \Delta E$.

Four tools developed in this research are available to the health economist that acts to advise a regulator.

1. A decision threshold that captures existing technical and allocative inefficiency and suboptimal displacement; the health shadow price, β_c.
2. A notation for the ICER of a new drug—the incremental price-effectiveness ratio (IPER)—that captures the endogeneity of the price of the drug to the pricing process.
3. Two metrics that allow that allow the firm's cost and profit functions for a new drug to be specified in terms of the incremental health effect of the new drug (the same units as the production function for the health budget):

   (a) The incremental cost of manufacturing an additional unit of effect of a new drug (IMER); and
   (b) The incremental economic rent of an additional unit of effect of a new drug (IπER).

4. Three examples of games that can be adapted to accommodate and assess any Threat claimed by a firm as part of a drug pricing process as the justification for maintaining a price above the decision threshold—and the contract that recognises the public's investment and return as a general solution to any version of this game.

And finally, four rules that should be followed by the regulator that chooses to play and win the new drug reimbursement game are identified.

1. Drug pricing is a game and the regulators make and enforce the rules.
2. Recognise that resources are constrained. If a new drug is reimbursed at an additional financial cost to the health budget, something, somewhere, will need to be displaced to finance it. It is likely that no health budget can be expanded to accommodate all purchases that are considered "value for money" in the lay sense of the term.[15]

---

[15] Without evidence of ICERs of all the health programs and technologies, this statement is difficult to prove. Certainly there are services that can be considered "cost ineffective" that are currently funded and could be disinvested. There are also other services that are cost-effective and that could be funded (Weinstein 2008). My point is simply that we cannot act as if health budgets are unconstrained, or are constrained only by some lay measure of "value for money" which is

3. Recognise that firms will act strategically. A rational firm will employ strategies to maximise their economic rent and the higher the potential rent the more a firm will invest into protecting or attracting that rent.
4. Never accept a price above the health shadow price without a contract with the firm that specifies the public's investment and return to the health budget.

1.7 Outline of Book

The book comprises three parts.

Part I provides background discussion on the political economy of new drugs, pharmaceutical innovation and its clinical and economic value. It begins with a discussion about political economy and its relevance to price of a new drug and the economic research that addresses this critical policy choice (Chap. 2). Chapter 3 presents a review of the "bottom line" empirical evidence supporting the current framing of the political economy of new drugs (PEND): (1) the high rate of return (in health gains) to investment in pharmaceutical R&D; and (2) increasing pharmaceutical R&D and new drugs as a major driver of the 10 year increase in the average life expectancy at birth of the US population from 1950 to 2009. The definition of the clinical value of innovation is clarified and distinguished from the term "pharmaceutical innovation", which applies to any new drug, regardless of its clinical advantages compared with either placebo or the best alternative therapy. Two additional types of pharmaceutical innovation are identified (Chap. 4). The significance of using a shadow price rather than a maxWTP to provide an economic value more generally is then demonstrated. Finally, a conventional method to derive the shadow price of an input or output when the market fails to provide a price is illustrated (Chap. 5).

Part II is concerned with the health economics of the choice of a threshold price for the reimbursement decision. The concepts of β_c and PEA are introduced. Part II starts with the derivation of β_c for the special case of an economically-efficient budget that is expanded to accommodate the additional cost of a new drug. PEA is introduced in Chap. 6 as a method used to characterise and quantify the relationship between price and population health outcomes. The capacity of β_c to capture information about variations in allocative and technical efficiency in the health

---

typically insensitive to changes in competition in the market for health inputs (See Chap. 3). Furthermore, an important theme in this book is that the choice of price by a firm that is a patent holder and has some monopoly power is endogenous to the choice of threshold; if a given threshold is imposed, firms with technologies that have ICERs greater than this threshold have the option to lower their price in order to make them "cost-effective". Therefore, technologies with ICERs greater than a given threshold will not necessary remain unfunded if that threshold is imposed (see Chap. 6). And finally, choice of a threshold needs to involve recognition of the budget constraint. Weinstein (2008) made a direct association between the US's preference for not applying CEA and decision thresholds and the lack of willingness of Americans to recognise they cannot Supply all citizens with "effective health care services".

budget and sub-optimality in displacement is demonstrated. In particular, its capacity to capture information about the strategy of improved allocative efficiency financed by optimal displacement as the best alternative strategy to reimbursement in an allocatively inefficient health budget is illustrated in Chap. 7. A simple applied game theoretic model is used to demonstrate the endogeneity of new drug price to the reimbursement process. This endogeneity concerns the relationship between new drug price and the institution's choice of decision threshold. This model predicts that as the threshold increases, so will a strategic profit-maximising firm's choice of the offer price per incremental effect of the new drug (Chap. 8).

Part III focuses on the pharma-economics of new drug price, in particular the question of whether the fact that the relationship between price and innovation is not captured by β_c means that the threshold price of the health effects of a new drug should be higher than β_c. Part III starts with two pharmaceutical industry cases for the FPP framed as specific threats and analysed within a game theoretic model and the PEA framework. Both of these threats are about how a price below the FPP is against the interests of the institution because it lowers the population's health. The two threats differ in terms of the mechanism underlying this claim. The first specific threat is a line of reasoning that links drug price and R&D funding via the failure of the capital market. Specifically:

• Firms rely on internal funds generated by above marginal cost pricing of new drugs because the capital markets fail to finance risky R&D. Hence without economic rents from higher prices it will not be possible to finance R&D.

This Game is called "The pharmaceutical R&D financing Game" (Chap. 9). The second specific threat is:

• Unless the decision threshold price of new drugs is given a premium over that applied to non-pharmaco-therapy, there will be less health in the future. Buying new drugs buys both current health and future health gain via innovation and the decision threshold must accommodate this.

This Game is called "The pharmaco-therapy needs a premium Game" (Chap. 10).

Chapter 11 presents the results of this research as a guide to regulators as to how to play and win the new drug reimbursement game. It presents the case for health economists to support the adoption of β_c as the decision threshold for the new drug reimbursement process. This case builds on the following observation: health economists have long questioned the practicality of using the opportunity cost of the additional cost of a new drug as the decision threshold price, primarily because of the absence of evidence of the opportunity cost. The starting point of an alternative approach to the political economy of the decision threshold is to ask why we do not have evidence of the best alternative strategy to new drug reimbursement and to identify β_c as a solution to this problem:

- In providing incentives for firms to develop evidence of the cost and effect of patented health technologies, institutions have failed to correct for the failure of the market to provide evidence of the cost and effect of unpatented or unpatentable health technologies and services. Using the β_c will provide an incentive for the institution to develop evidence of both the least and most cost-effective of currently funded programmes and hence correct for this market (and institutional) failure.

1.8 Playing and Winning the New Drug Reimbursement Game

If a regulator seeks to enforce the health shadow price as the maximum acceptable price, firms will respond with the Threat that lowering prices is against the interest of health funders because it will reduce a population's future health. The key to winning the new drug reimbursement game is to for the regulator to know how to respond to this Threat.

There are certain very restrictive conditions under which a population health maximising institution has an incentive to respond to this Threat by increasing the threshold price of a new drug above β_c. These conditions are identified in Chap. 10. Critically, the promise of clinical innovation from a future drug is found to be neither a necessary nor sufficient condition for a benefit to the population from higher prices and more future NMEs. A necessary condition is that the institution must contract with the firm to ensure that the institution can recoup the additional expenditure it makes today (higher prices), which will be invested into R&D by the firm. These funds are recouped through a discounted price of the future drug. It is highly likely that such a contract would be incomplete and unenforceable and hence it is uncertain whether the institution will reap the benefits in the future (more health gains than otherwise possible) of its investment today (higher drug prices means less funds for other inputs and less health effects from today's budget). This highly unlikely future benefit to the institution (and certain current net cost) is in contrast to the certainty that the firm will benefit from increased economic rent today. This benefit to the firm (more economic rent today) occurs regardless of whether this contract is enforced or the promise of a low cost future drug is an eventuality.

The most certain and significant consequence of a lower price today is a reduction in the firm's economic rent today. I conclude that, when the conditions are created for the institution to have an incentive to contract with the firm for higher prices today in return for more innovation in the future, it is in the interests of the firm to borrow from the capital market rather than the institution, if the former has a stronger preference for risk than the latter.

References

Birch S, Gafni A (1992) Cost effectiveness/utility analyses: do current decision rules lead us to where we want to be? J Health Econ 11(3):279–296

Birch S, Gafni A (1993) Changing the problem to fit the solution—Johannesson And Weinstein (mis) application of economics to real-world problems. J Health Econ 12(4):469–476

Buchanan J (2008) Opportunity cost. In: Durlauf S, Blume L (eds) The new Palgrave dictionary of economics online, 2nd edn. Palgrave Macmillian, New York. doi:10.1057/9780230226203. 1222

Canadian Coordinating Office for Health Technology Assessment (1994) Guidelines for economic evaluation of pharmaceuticals, 1st edn. CCOHTA, Ottawa, ON

Comanor W (1966) The drug industry and medical research: the economics of the Kefauver Committee investigations. J Bus 39(1):12–18

Comanor WS (1986) The political economy of the pharmaceutical industry. J Econ Lit 24 (3):1178–1217

Culyer A, McCabe C, Briggs A, Claxton K, Buxton M, Akehurst R, Sculpher M, Brazier J (2007) Searching for a threshold, not setting one: the role of the National Institute for Health and Clinical Excellence. J Health Serv Res Policy 12(1):56–58. doi:10.1258/135581907779497567

Devlin N, Parkin D (2004) Does NICE have a cost-effectiveness threshold and what other factors influence its decisions? A binary choice analysis. Health Econ 13(5):437–452

Drummond MF (1992) Basing prescription drug payment on economic analysis: the case of Australia. Health Aff (Millwood) 11:191–196

Finance Committee US Senate (2004) International trade and pharmaceuticals. Finance Committee US Senate, Washington, DC

George B, Harris A, Mitchell A (2001) Cost-effectiveness analysis and the consistency of decision making: evidence from pharmaceutical reimbursement in Australia (1991 to 1996). PharmacoEconomics 19(11):1103–1109

Giaccotto C, Santerre RE, Vernon JA (2005) Drug prices and research and development investment behavior in the pharmaceutical industry. J Law Econ 48(1):195–214

Gibbons RS (1992) A primer in game theory. Prentice Hall, Essex

Harvey K, Faunce T, Lokuge B, Drahos P (2004) Will the Australia–United States free trade agreement undermine the pharmaceutical benefits scheme? Med J Aust 181(5):256–259

International Trade Administration (2004) Pharmaceutical price controls in OECD countries: implications for U.S. consumers, pricing, research and development, and innovation. International Trade Administration, Washington, DC

Johannesson M, Weinstein MC (1993) On the decision rules of cost-effectiveness analysis. J Health Econ 12(4):459–467

McCabe C, Claxton K, Culyer AJ (2008) The NICE cost-effectiveness threshold: what it is and what that means. PharmacoEconomics 26(9):733

McKean RN (1972) The use of shadow prices. In: Layard R (ed) Cost benefit analysis. Penguin, Harmondsworth, pp 119–139

Mishan E, Quah E (2007) Cost-benefit analysis, 5th edn. Routledge, Abingdon

Reinhardt U (2007) The pharmaceutical sector in health care. In: Sloan F, Hsieh C-R (eds) Pharmaceutical innovation: incentives, competition, and cost-benefit analysis in international perspective. Cambridge University Press, Cambridge

Sager A (2003) Three futures for the US pharmaceutical industry. http://dcc2.bumc.bu.edu/hs/Upload061203/Sager%20talk%20Oxford%20-%20Chatham%2030%20May%2003%20final.pdf Accessed 12 Dec 2013

Sendi P, Gafni A, Birch S (2002) Opportunity costs and uncertainty in the economic evaluation of health care interventions. Health Econ 11(1):23–31

The National Institute for Health and Clinical Excellence (2007) Briefing paper for the methods working party on the cost effectiveness threshold. http://www.nice.org.uk/media/4A6/41/ CostEffectivenessThresholdFinalPaperTabledAtWPMeeting5Sep3907KT.pdf.   Accessed 12 Dec 2013

Vernon JA, Goldberg R, Golec JH (2009) Economic evaluation and cost-effectiveness thresholds: signals to firms and implications for R&D investment and innovation. PharmacoEconomics 27 (10):797–806

Weinstein MC (2008) How much are Americans willing to pay for a quality-adjusted life year? Med Care 46(4):343–345

Part I
The Political Economy of New Drugs and the Value of Pharmaceutical Innovation

Chapter 2
Reframing the Political Economy of New Drugs

Abstract The first rule of the new drug reimbursement game is to recognise it is a game and that the regulator makes the rules. The economic expression of this game is the Political Economy of New Drugs (PEND). The global PEND is driven and shaped primarily by the US: its pharmaceutical industry; its government via trade-negotiations with the Organisation for Economic Cooperation and Development (OECD); and US-based academic pharma-economists and the evidence they generate. In this chapter I use the PEND to illustrate the characteristics of this game. What is the political economy of new drugs? How does it influence the research agenda? Does it change over time? As the US starts to address issues such as whether it should use evidence of cost-effectiveness to make decisions about drug reimbursement, the global PEND must adapt to respond to the new forms of evidence and decision rules. I demonstrate how OECD regulators outside the US could use this time of change to reframe the global PEND. The reframed PEND would facilitate a strategic and economically meaningful choice in the decision threshold and allows regulators to respond optimally to the primary strategy of the pharmaceutical industry; the threat that lowering the price below a firm's preferred price is not in the best interests of the population.

2.1 The Political Economy of New Drugs

The term "Political Economy" is a former name of the discipline of economics. Today it is used in a number of senses, and its usage continues to evolve. Common to most of the modern interpretations is the economic analysis of tension in policy choices in a context that recognises both political and economic influences (Groenewegen 2008). In this book, the Political Economy of New Drugs (PEND) is defined following the precedent set by Comanor in his 1986 paper: "The Political Economy of the Pharmaceutical Industry". While Comanor did not explicitly define his use of this term, it can be inferred that the political economy of the pharmaceutical industry concerns the economics of the critical choices governments need to make about the pharmaceutical industry and its regulation. He identifies economics

© Springer International Publishing Switzerland 2015   21
B.A.K. Pekarsky, *The New Drug Reimbursement Game*,
DOI 10.1007/978-3-319-08903-4_2

as a "practical science" the practitioners of which have always been interested in the "critical choices" by governments.[1]

Of particular interest to Comanor was the relationship between the economist's research agenda and the politics of pharmaceutical regulation. He found that the political economy framed the research, and as the political debate changed so too did the research.

In this book the focus is "the political economy of new drugs": the factors that influence how any surplus associated with a new drug or a future drug is allocated across stakeholders, including consumers, purchasers, budget holders and firms.[2] The relationship between the economic research agenda and the political process identified by Comanor is also a central issue in this book. This book's focus on the political economy of new drugs rather than the pharmaceutical industry itself reflects the increased role of CEA in informing pricing and the capacity for industry, researchers and institutions to quantify the innovation associated with individual new drugs.

One way that the pharmaceutical industry seeks a share of a new drug's surplus is through lobbying. Lobbying plays an important part in the allocation of surplus associated with patented innovation in any sector of the economy. In the case of new drugs, lobbying tends to focus on the question of an appropriate price for a new drug, given the health-generating potential of both that drug and of future innovation funded by sales of the drug. The associated policy choices include: (1) whether new drug price should be regulated; (2) the selection of a decision threshold price in a reimbursement process; and (3) whether bilateral Free Trade Agreements (FTAs) with the US should be used by the US to prevent partner countries from regulating the price US firms prefer for their new drugs.

In the broader economy, lobbying by patent-holding firms is characterised as rent seeking or rent protection.[3] In the prevailing PEND, lobbying for higher new drug prices is instead characterised as providing incentives for investment into further R&D. This way of framing the impetus for lobbying links increased price to both increased profits and increased future health outcomes, thus creating an apparent win-win situation for firms and consumers. These claims of the relationship between new drug price and future health are supported by peer reviewed research and government studies (Comanor 1986; Scherer 2000; International

---

[1] See page 1178 in Comanor (1986).

[2] A UK example of the political economy of new drugs and the appropriation of surplus appears in a commentary on proposed changes to the UK pricing scheme (Towse 2007). Towse refers to the positive relationship between surplus appropriation by the innovator and the incentive for future innovation. Towse also recognises that if a higher share of this surplus is available to the health budget, immediate health gains increase. Towse also refers to the "high societal gains" from pharmaceuticals and new technologies but does not consider whether they are the best option available for improved future health gains nor does he consider how increasing the share appropriated by innovators impacts on the return to consumers.

[3] The term "rent seeking" was coined by Kruger and her original paper remains a significant milestone in the economics of lobbying and the associated deadweight social loss (Krueger 1974).

Trade Administration 2004; Vernon et al. 2009). This evidence base supports the claim that the relationship between price and R&D investment is positive and that new drugs are a key driver of improved longevity (life expectancy) for consumers.[4] The claim that firms rely on non-capital market-funded R&D rather than capital market borrowings due to the riskiness of this investment is supported by the pharma-economic literature.[5] The claim of and evidence for a win-win outcome to the policy of higher prices for new drugs is critical to the success of lobbying by US Pharma.

2.2   The Rate of Return on Investment in Pharmaceutical R&D and the Political Economy

Comanor argued that the political economy of the pharmaceutical industry shaped the economic research agenda, most notably the premise that there is a trade-off between savings today and health tomorrow: society can have more of one and less of the other but not more of both. Hence the purpose of much of the research was to quantify this trade-off. Comanor noted that the literature did not question whether this trade-off exists. Instead the research agenda prioritised finding an estimate of this trade-off, in the form of the ratio of the return (future health) on the original investment. Comanor identified three potentially relevant rates of return: the return to the firm in terms of economic rent from their investments; the return to the industry overall; and the social return, where return is measured as the increase in social welfare (economic rent and consumer welfare) from the investment in higher prices.

Comanor found that the focus on evidence of these rates of return was the single issue common to the disparate economic literature on the pharmaceutical industry. He also found that, at the time of his review (1986), no reliable estimate of the social rate of return on R&D had been published in the peer reviewed literature.[6] Comanor concluded that it could be possible to increase competition (lower price)

---

[4] While improved quality of life is also an outcome of improved pharmaco-therapy, the US literature and lobbying is dominated by the evidence supporting the claims of improved longevity at the population level. This situation is probably a consequence of the preference in the US economic literature for population based analysis of the benefits of pharmaceutical innovation rather than CEAs of individual new drugs. The complexity of measuring quality of life at the population level, without a control group, is far greater than that of measuring quality of life in a controlled clinical trial.

[5] "Non-capital market funded R&D" is a term used in this book to refer to the strategy by pharmaceutical firms of funding their investments in R&D through "internal funds" (economic rent) and publically financed health research such as the NIH (Vernon 2003; Keyhani et al. 2005; Santerre and Vernon 2006). This term distinguishes this strategy from the strategy of funding R&D by borrowing from the capital market.

[6] Comanor identified one study that estimated this return for three drugs but he found that the author had inflated this return by estimating the total social welfare from a given drug rather than the incremental social welfare from the innovation of this drug.

without having a loss in future innovation, however the current political economy excluded this possibility from the research agenda. Consequently, the evidence that could test this hypothesis (the possibility that there is no trade-off) was not available.

2.3   Is the Political Economy of New Drugs Constant?

Comanor observed that during the period from 1959 to 1985, the political economy of the pharmaceutical industry was reframed at least twice in response to changes in the political debate. The focus shifted from questioning whether the industry did in fact experience monopoly rents, to accepting that they did and then considering the impact of regulation on these rents and the incentive for R&D. Comanor also noted that the adversarial nature of the political debate was reflected in the economic research. He notes that at the start of economists' engagement with this political economy the focus was not on identifying critical trade-offs. Instead each side of the debate had a different premise, specifically, that the key issue was that competition should be restricted in order to maximise innovation and hence social welfare and the second ignoring this relationship.[7]

In the 25 years since Comanor's 1986 review of the political economy of the US pharmaceutical industry, the following have continued to grow: the US pharmaceutical industry[8]; US expenditure on pharmaceuticals and health as a percentage of Gross Domestic Product (GDP)[9]; the number of new drugs in the US development pipeline[10]; and the average longevity of the US population.[11] Studies have provided further evidence that the following relationships are positive: new drug price and

---

[7] See page 1180 in Comanor 1986.

[8] To the extent that the almost 50 % increase in expenditure on pharmaceuticals as a percent of GDP reflects growth in the US sector (see following footnotes), it is reasonable to surmise that the role of the US pharmaceutical sector as a percent of GDP has also increased since 1986. But how big was it in 2009? In 2009 an input output analysis of the US pharmaceutical sector prepared by consultants (Battelle Technology Partnership Practice) for the PhRMA (an industry lobby group formed by manufacturers that also conduct research) found that the output of the US biopharmaceutical sector represented 917B annually, with $382B in direct contribution (a multiplier of 2.4). Given that the US GDP was estimated at $14,043B this suggests that the pharmaceutical sector contributes (directly and indirectly) around 6.7 % of the total GDP and around 2.3 % for its direct contribution. It is in the interests of lobby groups to overestimate the role of their sector to the economy. For example, the authors write that: "A $10 billion change in US biopharmaceutical revenues would have the following effect on the U.S. economy: $29.7 billion in total output; 130,000 total jobs; $9.2 billion in personal income" PhRMA (2011).

[9] Total pharmaceutical expenditure increased from 8.8 % in 1986 to 12 % in 2009 Total Health expenditure increased from 10.6 % in 1986 to 17.4 % in 2009 (OECD Health Statistics 2013).

[10] From around 1,300 in 1997 to 2,995 in 2010 (PhRMA 2010).

[11] Life expectancy increased from 74.7 years at birth in 1986 to 78.2 in 2009 (OECD Health Statistics 2013).

R&D investment by firms (Vernon 2005); R&D investments and new drugs, as summarised by the costs of bring a new drug to market (DiMasi 2001); and new drugs and longevity (Lichtenberg 2006). Furthermore, other evidence suggests that the costs of bringing a new drug to market continues to increase as does society's demand for new drugs, particularly in relation to chronic diseases for which obesity is a risk factor (Grabowski et al. 2002; DiMasi et al. 2003).[12] The evidence supporting the case for higher new drug price appears to have strengthened, but the focus of evidence development has not broadened; the landscape of this political economy appears to have intensified but not shifted.

Since 1986, there have also been three main developments in the global pharmaceutical economy. First, institutions throughout the OECD started using formal processes such as HTA/CEA[13] to assess the incremental costs and benefits of new drugs compared with the best existing therapy.[14] The results of HTA/CEA are then used in conjunction with a decision threshold and other information to assess whether the population will be better or worse off if the institution reimbursed the drug at the firm's offer price. Hence, the policy debate throughout much of the OECD is increasingly broader than that of the US debate. The latter is primarily concerned with policies around discounts to large purchasers, whether there should be universal access to drugs, and whether HTA/CEA should be used and prices regulated. The rest of the OECD is additionally concerned with the choice of decision threshold and the type of information that should be included in an assessment of costs and benefits of new drugs.[15] However, the imperative to maximise the benefits of pharmaceutical and biotechnology innovation remains a significant part of OECD-wide research on pharmaceutical policy.[16]

---

[12] The proportion of the population who are obese, in the US increased from 23.3 % in 1991 to 33.8 % in 2008. These proportions are based on measured height and weight, not self-report, which tends to be lower. Obesity is defined as a $BMI > 30 \text{ kg/m}^2$ 2009 (OECD Health Statistics 2013).

[13] Chandra et al. (2011) describe cost-effectiveness analysis as "the half sibling to comparative analysis". The latter term appears to be used in the US in the same sense that HTA is used throughout counties that use economic evaluation.

[14] A summary of the range of OECD institutions that used economic evaluation in the mid 2000s is presented in ITA (2004). All countries have offices or institutions that place their local conventions in the public domain.

[15] Research such as that presented in Lakdawalla et al. (2009) is a good example of how the pharmaceutical policy issues faced by the US are far removed from the methodological debates that occupy countries such as the UK and the associated institutions such as National Institute for Health and Clinical Excellence (NICE). The commentary on this piece by the eminent pharmacoeconomist Scherer (2009) should be read in conjunction with that study; it summarises the technical reasons why their estimate of the health gains from new drugs are likely to be overestimates. The opinion piece by Weinstein (2008) shows how the US is still struggling with the question of whether or not they should use a CEA *at all* in decision making. Weinstein was a co-author of one of the seminal papers that sought to formalise CEA (Weinstein and Stason 1977). More than thirty years later, Weinstein (2008) observed that Americans still have not come to terms with the resource constraint in health care.

[16] For example see the policy document on the bioeconomy (OECD 2009).

Second, there has been a significant increase in the quantity of evidence about the relationship between: (1) price and innovation; and (2) new drugs in general and health.[17] However, it was only comparatively recently that the US pharma-economic literature provided two estimates of the ratio of the social return on consumers' investment in higher drug prices in the US. Lichtenberg's 2004 estimate of the social return on additional investment in new drug R&D is in the order of 160:1. Santerre and Vernon's (2006) estimate of a return on consumer's investment via higher prices over the period 1960–2000, in terms of the value of the additional health benefits from additional drugs, is in the order of 28:1.

Third, the US pharmaceutical industry now has two additional avenues to take the PEND to the rest of the OECD: (1) the formal reimbursement process for individual new drugs (lobbying for choice of decision threshold) (Vernon et al. 2010); and (2) the bilateral FTAs between the US and OECD countries (lobbying to prevent trading partners from regulating new drug price) (Harvey et al. 2004).

US pharma-economists have sought to adapt the original US political economy and research agenda to accommodate some of these changes. For example, Vernon et al. (2009) chose to define the socially optimal threshold from the perspective of optimal innovation. The authors started with the premise that socially optimal decision investment in R&D occurs when the firm can appropriate 100 % of the associated social surplus. Vernon et al. argue that this result occurs when the incremental cost per quality-adjusted life year (QALY) of a new drug is the same as the incremental cost per QALY of the least cost-effective of currently funded services. The authors argue this reference is the provision of dialysis at a cost per QALY of $129,000. Other authors have argued that setting a price threshold of i[18] and comparing the results of CEA against this threshold of i is price control under another name and its result is the same: pricing below the free market price will lead to a deadweight social loss.[19] Jena and Philipson have published a number of papers about the inclusion of dynamic welfare considerations in the decision threshold (Jena and Philipson 2007, 2008). Originally they argued that this threshold should be the maxWTP, just as Vernon et al. have claimed. Their rationale included that "technology adoption through cost-effectiveness is a price-control policy in disguise and might therefore have many of the properties of such policies." However, in the later paper they recognised a number of factors that supported the case for the threshold to be lower than the maxWTP. These factors include budget constraints and the contribution by public sector research funds to pharmaceutical R&D. Jena and Philipson did not specify exactly what this price should be, only that it should be higher than the threshold applied to non-pharmacological therapies.

---

[17] Sloan and Hsieh provide a comprehensive summary of this literature (Sloan and Hsieh 2007).

[18] For example, $75,000 per incremental QALY.

[19] For example, the report on OECD price controls prepared by the US International Trade Administration (2004).

One key aspect of the political economy has remained constant, despite these developments: the trade-off between savings today and health tomorrow remains the central premise.[20] The possibility that increased competition (lower prices) could lead to more health in the future as well as today is not part of the research agenda. Furthermore, it is a possibility that continues to be excluded from the prevailing political economy.

2.4 Reframing the Political Economy

- Is it possible to reframe rather than adapt the prevailing PEND to accommodate the developments in drug reimbursement and HTA/CEA?
- Could this reframed political economy include the possibility that each of the following can be simultaneously improved: competition; current health; and future health?

This reframed political economy would focus on the central policy decision by a reimbursing institution: which decision threshold will maximise the npvPH? The first step in this research was to develop a formal model to define the political economy of new drugs in the context of policy choice and research. The model was used to specify both the current and alternative frames for the political economy.

2.4.1 Architecture of Evidence Based Policy

The relationship between the PEND and the research agenda is characterised using an adaption of Grüne-Yanoff and Schweinzer's Architecture of Game Theory (Grüne-Yanoff and Schweinzer 2008) with additional elements derived from Roe (1991) and Comanor (1986). The adaption is described in Pekarsky (2012, Appendix 1) and illustrated in Fig. 2.1. Amongst other advantages, this framework identifies the line of reasoning that leads to certain possibilities being excluded from the prevailing research agenda. For example, by defining the key trade-off as being between more health tomorrow and more savings today, the possibility that both competition and population health can be improved is excluded. Consequently, this framework identifies that there is a requirement to redefine the evidence based policy framework that shapes the current research agenda and suggests some mechanisms by which this could be achieved.

The following two sections populate this framework, first with a characterisation of the prevailing political economy and the second with an alternative frame.

---

[20] This is also expressed as the trade-off between access today and health tomorrow (Scherer 2000) and decreased welfare of current patients due to higher prices and increased welfare of future patients due to more innovation from these higher prices (Jena and Philipson 2007).

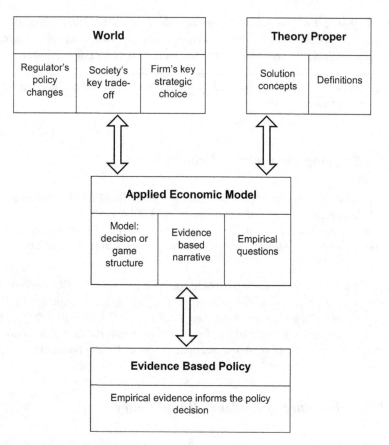

Fig. 2.1 An architecture of applied economics

2.4.2 Prevailing Political Economy

The key *trade-off* is between savings today and health tomorrow, for example:

- If the price of today's new drug is reduced below the FPP, there will be financial savings for *some* today but this is at the cost of access to more drugs for the *whole population* in the future.[21]

---

[21] An excerpt from the Joint Hearing of the Finance Committee of the US Senate in April 2004 is reproduced in Attachment 2 and contains a number of variations of this theme. This characterisation is a synthesis of the extensive literature on this topic, much of which is summarised in Comanor (1986) and Scherer (2000). Specific examples include: "Greater access to today's medicines... through drug price controls at a cost of fewer new drugs in the future" and "Understanding this tradeoff is imperative for sound public policy." (Vernon 2004). Another example is Vernon et al.'s (2006) analysis of a change in pricing policy in the US in which the authors state that the policy debate on lower prices should consider the "hidden potential costs" of lower prices (less innovation). They state that their analysis does not provide evidence of the "relative costs and benefits of pharmaceutical importation (or price regulation)." But then go on to infer that these "hidden potential costs" are so significant that they dominate policy choices.

The key *decision by the firm* is how much to invest in R&D and the key *policy choice* is whether or not to regulate or control the new drug price. This particular framing inspires *research questions* such as:

- What is the relationship between today's price of a new drug, pharmaceutical R&D and future innovation? (Vernon 2005; Abbott and Vernon 2007; Vernon et al. 2009); and
- What is the incentive for purchasers to maintain prices at the FPP? (Lichtenberg 2004; Santerre and Vernon 2006).

This frame excludes empirical questions about the direction of the relationship between: (1) new drug price, R&D, number of new drugs; and (2) future health of the population. This relationship is assumed to be positive under all conditions. The *critical piece of information* that will inform the regulator is the return on this investment in R&D (financed via higher prices and public investment), where this return is measured as the additional health gains possible from the availability of additional drugs in the future. If the health effects are monetised, for example using an estimate of the value of an additional year of life, then the return can be compared to the investment as a ratio. If this ratio is high then increased prices today represent a good evidence-based policy choice. If this ratio is less than one, then there is a net loss on the original investment.

The *evidence-based policy narrative* takes the following or a related form.

New drugs have been shown to be the key driver of historic gains in life expectancy for the US population. In order to achieve sustained increases in life expectancy, more new drugs are needed in the future. Pharmaceutical innovation is driven by R&D investments by firms. R&D investments are driven by higher new drug prices, acting as both an incentive and a funding source for ongoing R&D. The value of the possible health gains far outweigh the financial costs of R&D, therefore higher—unregulated—prices represent good policy.

2.4.3 An Alternative Political Economy of New Drugs

This book explores the fresh paths for research and different critical research questions opened by reframing the prevailing PEND. There are many ways that the political economy could be reframed. The frame used in this book is summarised as follows.

The key *trade-off* is between savings for health purchasers today and firms' profits. The evidence for this trade-off is twofold. First, a firm would not lobby for a higher price unless this strategy increased its profits in the current period. Second, an institution would not reject a higher price of new drugs if it also decreased costs of providing the same health benefits from today's budget. Therefore the existence of this trade-off is a reasonable premise.

The key *decision by the firm* is how to maximise profits today and tomorrow. One strategy available to the firm is to minimise the R&D costs borne by the firm by creating an incentive for institutions to subsidise these costs. One mechanism by which this is achieved is to increase the price of current drugs, without reducing quantity sold (for example, increase the decision threshold). The key *policy choices* for the institution are: (1) what should the decision threshold for the health effects for new drugs be; and (2) should this threshold be altered, given that there is a relationship between new drug price today and future population health. This particular framing inspires *research questions* such as:

- Given that budgets are constrained or fixed, under what conditions will increased pharmaceutical R&D today necessarily lead to increased population health in the future?;
- What about the impact on the population's future health due to less resources being allocated to health care today?; and
- How should institutions respond to Pharma's strategy of lobbying to increase the decision threshold?

The *critical pieces of information* for the institution are: (1) what is the maximum acceptable price for new drugs; and (2) how does this maximum price change if there is a relationship between price and the npvPH. The *evidence-based narrative* takes the following or a related form.

> Higher prices today mean increased economic rent for Pharma otherwise they would not lobby for them. It is in Pharma's interest to protect and seek these economic rents. Whether higher prices and more R&D today increase future health remains an empirical question. If higher prices also mean a higher net present value of the population's health, then it is in the institution's interest to increase prices. Given the institution's objectives, the most effective strategy a firm can use to protect these rents is "the Threat": lowering prices is against the interest of health funders because it will reduce a population's future health.

In this alternative framing, the market within which pharmaceuticals compete is expanded to include any health input, including unpatented programs and technologies. Competition for pharmaceutical R&D funds would include investments in other forms of medical and health innovation, including those that cannot be patented, and research on workforce and service delivery. The reframed political economy also recognises that there is a failure by markets to provide evidence of the cost-effectiveness of unpatented and unpatentable programmes. It recognises firms' rent-seeking motives, accepts these as rational, and explicates the increased rent available to firms as a consequence of lobbying. Finally, it includes both of the following possible consequences of increased price of new drugs today, not just the first (as is the case with the prevailing political economy):

- New drug prices increase and the future health of the population improves; and
- New drug prices increase and the health of the current and future populations decreases.

Consequently, the following two central premises of the prevailing political economy become testable hypotheses under this alternative framing:

- Higher drug prices, more R&D and more new future drugs will always increase the future health of the population; and
- There is a trade-off between savings (and additional health from improved access) today[22] and health tomorrow.

2.4.4 Comparison of Prevailing and Proposed Frames

The prevailing and alternative frames of the political economy are compared Tables 2.1, 2.2, 2.3 and 2.4 in relation to each four components: World; Applied Economic Model; Theory; and Evidence Based Decisions. Only the alternative frame accommodates the possibility that the health of the future population might increase or decrease as a consequence of lower drug prices today. The alternative frame is designed to find the solution to the following policy problem: the choice of a decision threshold price for new drugs, where this threshold accommodates both characteristics of the health budget and the relationship between price today and innovation in the future. This intent is in contrast to the prevailing frame, which, as demonstrated in Chap. 3 and Pekarsky (2012, Appendix 7) is specified so as to fit a particular solution. This solution is that threshold prices below the firm's preferred price or the maxWTP are not in the interest of an institution seeking to maximise the population's health (1993).[23]

One issue that is raised by this alternative political economy is that it is not possible to calculate the critical ratio of costs to benefits of lower prices without evidence of the counterfactual. The counterfactual to higher drug prices becomes

---

[22] The reference to reduction in health today as a consequence of increased expenditure on more costly drugs was originally part of this trade-off. Typically this was expressed as the trade-off between access (lower priced drugs so that everyone, particularly the uninsured could afford them) and more health in the future. See for example Scherer (2000). However, increasingly the US literature expresses this as a trade-off between savings today and health in the future. For example, see Santerre and Vernon (2006). The critical question then is to compare the financial value of future health effects against these savings. For reasons discussed and demonstrated in Chap. 3, this particular framing results in a higher ratio of the gains in the future compared to the loss today.

[23] The contrast between framing a problem to "find" rather than "fit" the solution comes from Birch and Gafni (1993).

Table 2.1 Reframing the political economy of new drugs: World

	Framing the problem to FIT the solution	Framing the problem to FIND the solution
Trade-off	Savings today vs. more health in the future population	More economic rent today vs. more health (or more savings) today
Firm strategies	How much to invest in the R&D for new drugs?	How much to invest in lobbying for a higher price?
	What is the price at which R&D is optimised?	What is the most effective way to increase and protect economic rent?
Regulator policies	Should the new drug price be controlled?	What is the decision threshold (shadow price) for the additional health effect a new drug?
	How much should the public sector invest in R&D?	How much to invest in the development of evidence of counterfactuals?
	How should FTAs accommodate pharmaceutical pricing?	How to respond to the threat that lower prices are not in the population's interest?

Table 2.2 Reframing the political economy of new drugs: applied economic model

	Framing the problem to FIT the solution	Framing the problem to FIND the solution
Evidence based narrative	Improved longevity is driven by Pharma R&D. To continue to improve longevity we need to continue invest in R&D via higher prices and more public research funds	Less than 30 % of the economic rent from higher prices is allocated to NME R&D. Firms have an incentive to generate and protect these rents. The most effective threat is to claim that the higher prices are in the interest of the population's health
Model structure	Decision theoretic, uncertainty but no private information and new drug price is exogenous to the reimbursement process	Game theoretic, assuming that there is strategic response, new drug price is endogenous to the reimbursement process and firms hold private information (information in their private domain)
Research questions	What is the health value of historic R&D decisions?	What is the economic value of the clinical innovation of new drugs?
	What is the response of R&D to new drug price?	How much to invest in developing evidence of counterfactuals to Pharma R&D?
	What is the health return on consumers' investment in R&D?	Under what conditions will a price above the shadow price increase the npvPH?

Table 2.3 Reframing the political economy of new drugs: theory

	Framing the problem to FIT the solution	Framing the problem to FIND the solution
Theory proper	Firms require the full surplus associated with the drug in order to achieve socially optimal levels of R&D. Price control leads to a deadweight social loss and pharmaceutical price control is no exception to this basic economic fact	Shadow price of new drugs should accommodate existing inefficiencies and all alternative investment opportunities by the public sector. Firms have private information. There is a failure of markets to develop evidence of unpatentable health innovation

Table 2.4 Reframing the political economy of new drugs: Evidence based decisions

	Framing the problem to FIT the solution	Framing the problem to FIND the solution
Evidence	New drugs have contributed significantly to improvements in US longevity that would not have occurred without this R&D	The improvements in longevity experienced in the US are below those experienced in other countries such as Canada, UK and Australia. [See Pekarsky (2012, Appendix 3)] These other countries have not corrected for the failure of the market to provide evidence of the counterfactual but they have provided incentives to develop evidence of the cost and effect of new drugs
	There is a return of 28-fold in health benefits from every dollar invested in R&D raised through higher new drug price	
Policy decisions	Do not regulate new drug price	It could be that there is a price above the shadow price that is better for the npvPH. If this is the case, this price should be adopted. Otherwise the shadow price should be applied. How much should be invested to correct for the markets failure to generate evidence of unpatented and unpatentable services, technologies and programs?
	Increase public subsidy of private Pharma R&D	
	Use FTAs to control regulation in other countries	

relevant when the budget is assumed to be either fixed or constrained (that is, not unconstrained). (See the discussion of these terms in Sect. 3.3.) However, without evidence of the alternative uses of these funds, it is not possible to determine whether or not a country such as the US could have done better by investing in alternative technologies (perhaps with a low ICER) or in unpatented programmes. This issue is also relevant to countries that use HTA/CEA to inform new drug adoption decisions. The pharma-economic literature is strongly supportive of the use of patents to generate a financial incentive for investing in the R&D for new drugs. However, as Arrow (1962) and Tirole (1988) both conclude, the failure of the market to provide an incentive to invest in innovation where that innovation cannot be patented is an economic case for public sector investment. The failure of the market to provide an incentive to invest in developing evidence of unpatented programmes and technologies is not afforded the same attention by pharma-economists as the potential failure to protect the results of patentable, pharmaceutical R&D (Sloan and Hsieh 2007). The issue of absence of evidence of the counterfactual is a barrier to testing the key empirical question under the prevailing frame. In the alternative frame, the absence of this evidence is a characteristic of economic context; the failure of the market to provide evidence of the unpatented counterfactual to higher prices.

2.5   Conclusion

The global PEND shapes the pharma-economic research agenda. But how can we reframe the political economy and research agenda so as to accommodate the critical policy issues faced by institutions outside the US? There is more than one way this alternative political economy could be specified. The frame proposed in this chapter and used throughout this book has a number of features that distinguish it from the prevailing political economy. One of these features is that it recognises that there is that pharmaceuticals face competition in the market for health inputs, including competition from unpatented and unpatentable technologies and inputs. Consequently, a critical piece of evidence is a qualitative value (equation) of a health shadow price that reflects the competition in the market for health inputs.

In the alternative PEND the evidence of the historic rate of return on consumers' investment in pharmaceutical R&D via higher prices is no longer the key piece of evidence that informs policy. However, if the evidence provided by Santerre and Vernon (2006) and Lichtenberg (2004) that this return is very high (between 28 and 160 for each dollar of higher prices) is correct, then it would appear that the value of an alternative political economy that can also identify the possibility of an increase in current and future health from lower prices is limited; it will not change a policy decision.

In the following chapter, I show that despite the US evidence of a very high ratio of social return on pharmaceutical R&D, it is both possible and plausible that, had prices of new drugs in the US been lower over the past 50 years, that the health of the US population today could have been better. A high return, as calculated in the US literature, does not exclude the possibility that lower prices can improve current and future health.

References

Abbott TA, Vernon JA (2007) The cost of US pharmaceutical price regulation: a financial simulation model of R&D decisions. Manag Decis Econ 28(4–5):293–306

Arrow KJ (1962) Economic welfare and the allocation of resources for invention. In: National Bureau of Economic Research (ed) The Rate and direction of inventive activity: economic and social factors—a conference of the Universities. Princeton University Press, Princeton, NJ

Birch S, Gafni A (1993a) Changing the problem to fit the solution: Johannesson and Weinstein's (mis) application of economics to real-world problems. J Health Econ 12(4):469–476

Chandra A, Jena A, Skinner J (2011) The Pragmatist's guide to comparative effectiveness research. J Econ Perspect 25(2):27–46

Comanor WS (1986) The political economy of the pharmaceutical industry. J Econ Lit 24 (3):1178–1217

DiMasi JA (2001) New drug development in the United States from 1963 to 1999. Clin Pharmacol Ther 69(5):286–296

DiMasi JA, Hansen RW, Grabowski HG (2003) The price of innovation: new estimates of drug development costs. J Health Econ 22(2):151–185

Grabowski H, Vernon J, DiMasi JA (2002) Returns on research and development for 1990s new drug introductions. PharmacoEconomics 20:11–29

Groenewegen P (2008) Political economy. In: Durlauf SN, Blume LE (eds) The New Palgrave dictionary of economics. Palgrave Macmillan, Basingstoke

Grüne-Yanoff T, Schweinzer P (2008) The roles of stories in applying game theory. J Econ Methodol 15(2):131–146

Harvey K, Faunce T, Lokuge B, Drahos P (2004) Will the Australia–United States free trade agreement undermine the pharmaceutical benefits scheme? Med J Aust 181(5):256–259

International Trade Administration (2004) Pharmaceutical price controls in OECD countries: implications for U.S. consumers, pricing, research and development, and innovation. Department of Commerce, Washington, DC

Jena AB, Philipson TJ (2007) Cost-effectiveness as a price control. Health Aff 26(3):696–703

Jena AB, Philipson TJ (2008) Cost-effectiveness analysis and innovation. J Health Econ 27:1224–1236

Keyhani S, Diener-West M, Powe N (2005) Do drug prices reflect development time and government investment? Med Care 43(8):753–762

Krueger A (1974) The political economy of the rent-seeking society. Am Econ Rev 64(3):291–303

Lakdawalla DN, Goldman DP, Michaud P-C, Sood N, Lempert RJ, Cong Z, de Vries H, Gutierrez I (2009) U.S. pharmaceutical policy in a global marketplace. Health Aff 28(1):w138–w150

Lichtenberg FR (2004) Sources of U.S. longevity increase, 1960-2001. Q Rev Econ Finance 44 (3):369–389

Lichtenberg FR (2006) Pharmaceutical innovation and the longevity of Australians: a first look. http://www.cfses.com/documents/events/Lichtenberg_2007_Pharmaceutical_innovation_&_ longevity.pdf Accessed 25 Dec 2013

OECD (2009) The Bioeconomy to 2030: designing a policy agenda. http://www.oecd.org/futures/ bioeconomy/2030. Accessed Dec 2013

OECD Health Statistics (2013) Organisation for economic co-operation and development. www. oecd.org Accessed 25 Dec 2013

Pekarsky BAK (2012) Trust, constraints and the counterfactual: reframing the political economy of new drug price. Dissertation, University of Adelaide. http://digital.library.adelaide.edu.au/ dspace/handle/2440/79171. Accessed 25 Dec 2013

PhRMA (2010) U.S. Market Drives Global Development of Medicines. http://www.phrma.org/us-market-drives-global-development-medicines Accessed 25 Dec 2013

PhRMA (2011) The biopharmaceuticals sector: the economic contribution to a nation. http://www. phrma.org/sites/default/files/159/2011_battelle_report_on_economic_impact.pdf. Accessed 25 Dec 25 2013

Roe E (1991) Development narratives, or making the best of blueprint development. World Dev 19(4):287–300

Santerre RE, Vernon JA (2006) Assessing consumer gains from a drug price control policy in the United States. South Econ J 73(1):233–245

Scherer FM (2000) The pharmaceutical industry. In: Culyer AJ, Newhouse JP (eds) Handbook of health economics volume 1 A, vol 17, Handboooks in economics. Elsevier, Amsterdam, pp 1297–1336

Scherer FM (2009) Price controls and global pharmaceutical progress. Health Aff 28(1):w161–w164

Sloan FA, Hsieh C-R (2007) Conclusions and policy implications. In: Sloan FA, Ruey HC (eds) Pharmaceutical innovation: incentives, competition, and cost-benefit analysis in international perspective. Cambridge University Press, New York, pp 262–277

Tirole J (1988) The theory of industrial organization. MIT, Cambridge, MA

Towse A (2007) If it ain't broke, don't price fix it: the OFT and the PPRS. Health Econ 16 (7):653–665

Vernon JA (2003) Price regulation, capital market imperfections, and strategic R&D investment behavior in the pharmaceutical industry: consequences for innovation. University of Pennsylvania, Philadelphia, PA

Vernon JA (2004) Pharmaceutical R&D investment and cash flows: an instrumental variables approach to testing for capital market imperfections. J Pharm Finance Econ Policy 13(4):3–17

Vernon JA (2005) Examining the link between price regulation and pharmaceutical R&D investment. Health Econ 14(1):1–16

Vernon JA, Golec JH, Hughen WK (2006) The economics of pharmaceutical price regulation and importation: refocusing the debate. Am J Law Med 32(2–3):175–192

Vernon JA, Goldberg R, Golec JH (2009) Economic evaluation and cost-effectiveness thresholds: signals to firms and implications for R & D investment and innovation. PharmacoEconomics 27(10):797–806

Vernon JA, Golec JH, Stevens JS (2010) Comparative effectiveness regulations and pharmaceutical innovation. PharmacoEconomics 28(10):877–887

Weinstein MC (2008) How much are Americans willing to pay for a quality-adjusted life year? Med Care 46(4):343–345

Weinstein MC, Stason WB (1977) Foundations of cost-effectiveness analysis for health and medical practices. N Engl J Med 296(13):716–721

Chapter 3
The Social Rate of Return on Investment in Pharmaceutical Research and Development

Abstract The conventional method of assessing the value of higher prices of new drugs is the ratio of investment in research and development (R&D) sourced from internal funds to the additional health for the population due to additional future New Molecular Entities (NMEs). There is evidence that the conventionally defined ratio is significantly greater than one. But does this mean that higher prices are necessarily in the population's interest? A positive correlation between additional future NMEs and future health for the population is a central premise of the prevailing political economy of new drug price. In this chapter I show that a positive correlation is not axiomatic; it is a testable hypothesis and its direction depends on the economic context of the health budget. I present a general expression for the estimate of a return on increased drug prices and public funding for private pharmaceutical R&D that accommodates this context. I distinguish between three types of health budget constraints: (1) a fixed budget that cannot be expanded; (2) a constrained budget that can be expanded incrementally, but only by foregoing the best alternative strategy; and (3) an unconstrained budget that expands to fund every programme that is "cost-effective" in the lay sense of the term. I use this general expression to show that if the health budget is constrained or fixed, even a very high ratio of conventionally defined return to investment does not exclude the possibility that today's health could have been better had historic prices and R&D been lower.

3.1 The Reimburser's Problem

A country with a universal health care system and a fixed budget is negotiating a FTA with the US. During the negotiation a US senator visits the country and explains that, even though he is advocating on behalf of the US government, he also has the interest of the citizens of this country at heart. He argues that the evidence is clear; increased life expectancy is driven by new medicines and the availability of new medicines is driven by more pharmaceutical R&D, which is in turn driven by not regulating the FPP. Citizens in all countries would be better off if countries like this one stopped regulating the FPP. The short-term gain of financial

© Springer International Publishing Switzerland 2015
B.A.K. Pekarsky, *The New Drug Reimbursement Game*,
DOI 10.1007/978-3-319-08903-4_3

savings would be at the cost of the population's longer-term health; higher prices mean more health.

The Minister for Health and the Minister for International Trade ask the Reimburser her opinion as to whether applying a decision threshold price per effect for new drugs that is lower than the FPP will lead the population's health to be worse off in the longer run. (The Reimburser makes the final decision regarding the adoption of a new drug at its offer price based on evidence of its additional cost and effect.) The Reimburser is provided with evidence of the gain in average life expectancy at birth in the US; a gain of a full decade over the 60 years from 1950 to 2009. She is also provided with a summary of the peer reviewed evidence of the significance of the contribution of new medicines to this gain (PhRMA 2011). This report concludes that the contribution of new drugs to increased life expectancy in areas such as HIV and cardiovascular disease is in the order of 50–80 %.

The Reimburser is also presented with a study that estimates that the health return on consumer investment in R&D via higher prices (foregone consumer surplus) in the US between 1960 and 2000 is in the order of 28:1 (Santerre and Vernon 2006). A study by Lichtenberg estimates that the social return on pharmaceutical R&D over 1960–2001 was in the order of 160:1 (Lichtenberg 2004). Furthermore, in the concluding chapter of a recent text on the topic of pharmaceutical innovation with contributions from a range of eminent pharma-economists, the editors write that give the evidence suggests that returns are in the order of 10 to 1 that the cost at which developed countries have achieved better health through drugs is much less than the value of this longevity gain.[1]

Finally, the Reimburser is given a study by Lichtenberg that explores the relationship between drug vintage (the years since patent granted) and Australian improvements in mean age at death and other variables. This study concluded that because their calculations suggest that of the 2 year gain in life expectancy in Australia in the 8 years to 2003, 65 % is attributable to new drugs, that 1.3 (two thirds of 2 years) of this life expectancy would otherwise not have occurred.[2]

As intuitively appealing as this line of reasoning is, the Reimburser is unsure whether it is sufficient to justify a policy of increased prices of new drugs via a higher threshold. She has these concerns, even though the purported objective of such a policy is the same as the Reimburser's objective that is, increasing the population's health. She performs a rough calculation of the estimated additional financial cost to the pharmaceutical budget of the proposed increase in price for new drugs for the next year; a 10 % increase in the pharmaceutical budget. The Reimburser then realises that the additional financial cost to the pharmaceutical budget is permanent; it is not a one-off increase in prices but a policy that would lead to all future pharmaceutical budgets being higher than would otherwise be the case. Furthermore, the policy is expected to lead to more new drugs in the future than would otherwise be the case and they will all be at this higher new price. These

---

[1] See page 273 in Sloan and Hsieh (2007).

[2] See page 14 in Lichtenberg and Duflos (2008).

additional costs will need to be financed somehow; because the current fiscal climate is one of restraint, other programmes will need to be displaced in order to accommodate these additional costs. While there might be $28 worth of health benefits to certain *patients* for every additional dollar invested in R&D via higher prices, the ratio of additional *population* health to additional R&D dollars could be much smaller, or even negative.[3] Even if the budget is increased to accommodate these additional costs, other programmes, including the extension of existing programmes, will be foregone. Lichtenberg's conclusion that the increase in average longevity of a population that is attributable to new drugs would not have occurred in the absence of these drugs is only reasonable under a very restrictive condition: had these new drugs not been purchased from the budget at the higher cost, and older drugs used instead, the savings could not be used to purchase any other services other than drugs that would have also contributed to life expectancy gains.

The Reimburser reviews the US evidence. It seems to her that the basis upon which this return on R&D is estimated makes no reference to these foregone opportunities.[4] Can the US pharma-economists and regulators conclude, as they routinely do, that the US population would have been worse off with lower drug prices, if they have not considered the evidence of foregone benefits—the counterfactual? If this evidence of the counterfactual is made available and is found to support the case for higher prices of drugs in the US, can the US trade negotiators claim that all countries will be better off with unregulated (higher) drug prices? The Reimburser wonders if her intuition about the limitations of this evidence has an economic foundation.

The Reimburser asks her Health Economic Adviser:

- Does the US estimate of a 28-fold health return on pharmaceutical R&D financed by higher drug prices exclude the possibility that at lower prices and fewer NMEs the US population's longevity would now be even higher?

---

[3] This would be the case if the additional services displaced to finance the additional new drugs had a lower ICER compared to the ICER of the new drugs.

[4] A review of this literature is presented in Pekarsky (2012, Appendix 2). The summary presented in this chapter is primarily concerned with evidence of the social return to consumers' investment in Pharma R&D via higher prices.

3.2   A Closer Look at the Evidence Supporting Pharma's Lobbying

3.2.1   Why Is Return on Consumers' Investment in Pharmaceutical R&D Important?

US Pharma sources the majority of its funds for R&D from non-capital market funding: purchasers (via higher prices) and public and private not-for-profit research institutes (Joint Economic Committee 2000; Lichtenberg 2004; Giaccotto et al. 2005). Therefore, US Pharma must lobby (rather than contract with the capital market) to ensure that these funds are at least ongoing, if not increasing. While there is no doubt that increased economic rent for Pharma is an objective of this lobbying for higher price, this is not a politically or socially acceptable justification for non-capital market investment (higher prices). In simple terms, Pharma cannot lobby for higher prices using the following justification: "increase prices because, even though it will increase your organisation's costs, it will increase our profits". Instead Pharma must lobby on the basis that there is a return to the funder of this additional R&D, namely, an increase in the population's future health.

Comanor (1986) observed that the single feature uniting the disparate US pharma-economic literature from the 1959 Kefauver Committee[5] to the publication of Comanor's paper in 1986 was the recognition that the most critical piece of information in the current political economy was an estimate of the return on this investment in pharmaceutical R&D. Comanor also noted three ways in which this return on R&D was defined: the return to the individual firms, the return to the industry and the social return in terms of improved health. It is the last of these three that is of particular interest to the Reimburser and other purchasers and to public health research funding bodies as providers of funds to finance the R&D.

At the time of Comanor's 1986 publication, no estimate of the social return existed. Comanor reported that one study (Wu and Lindgren 1984) had found social rates of return on three specific new products' R&D of 65 %, 169 % and 69 %. However, Comanor noted that the study had not deducted "the consumer and producer surpluses obtained from predecessor products" and that "this lead to inflated values".[6]

Comanor also noted a practice by US pharma-economists of inferring that the costs of regulation outweighed "any prospective benefits at the regulatory margin". In simple terms, when some economists identified that there was an unintended negative consequence of increased regulation, they would infer (not prove) that this cost outweighed the benefits of that regulation. For example, increasing the amount

---

[5] See footnote 2, Chap. 1.

[6] This is analogous to calculating the clinical value of innovation by comparing it to placebo rather than the best available existing care. This approach results in an overestimate of the clinical innovation of a new drug, where this overestimate increases as the clinical innovation of the comparator increases (see Chap. 2).

of evidence about a new drug that needs to be reviewed by a regulator such as the Food and Drug Administration (FDA) will have the intended consequence of improving safety, but with the unintended consequence of forgone health effects due to the delay in the time for new drugs to reach the market (International Trade Administration 2004 p. 6). Therefore, some pharma-economists might infer that this leads to a net social loss. Comanor identified that the issue is whether the net consequences (identified and unintended) outweigh the benefits that regulation—not simply whether there are unintended consequences.[7]

If the evidence of the social rate of return, the major justification of ongoing non-capital market investment in R&D, was not available in 1986 then when did it become available?

3.2.2   What Is the Evidence of the Return on Consumers' Investment?

3.2.2.1   A Review of the Literature

Numerous US pharma-economic studies published between 2000 and 2010 conclude or infer that the result of their study supports the policy of allowing drug companies to price without regulation because society's return on increased pharmaceutical R&D is high and therefore a population's future health will be worse if the price of drugs is lowered. However, a detailed review of these studies[8] revealed that only two published studies attempted to provide the evidence that is required to inform this policy choice (the return from pharmaceutical R&D estimated as a social return on non-capital market investment). These studies are Santerre and Vernon (2006) and Lichtenberg (2004). So what evidence do these other studies, all of which refer to this return, actually provide?

The remaining studies included in the review were classified into three groups. The first group, which included most of the remaining studies, provided evidence that supports the "policy narrative", but not the policy choice. The evidence that supports the policy narrative is wide ranging. Some studies indicate that if profit increases, so too does investment in R&D (Vernon 2004). Other studies provide evidence of the high and increasing present value of the costs of bringing a new drug to market (DiMasi et al. 2003). One study demonstrated that even the threat of price control in the US was sufficient to reduce R&D investment (Golec et al. 2005). The second group of studies provided evidence of rate of return estimates for the purchase of new drugs (not drug R&D). For example, retrospective analysis of historic data showed that increased expenditure on new drugs led to a health benefit with a monetary value greater than the additional cost of these drugs

---

[7] See page 1207 in Comanor (1986).

[8] This review is presented in Pekarsky (2012, Appendix 2).

(Cremieux et al. 2007).[9] The third group comprised three studies which could, under very restrictive conditions, be interpreted as providing evidence of the social rate of return; however, these conditions were very unlikely to occur.

3.2.2.2   The Two Published Estimates of the Social Return to Consumers' Investment in High Prices

The two studies published between 2000 and 2010 that estimated a return on the ongoing non-capital market investment in pharmaceutical R&D found a very high return on historic investments of consumer surplus in pharmaceutical R&D via higher prices; in the order of 28-fold from Santerre and Vernon's study and 160-fold from Lichtenberg's study. These estimates of return are a powerful piece of evidence supporting continued and increased investment in pharmaceutical R&D via non-capital market sources. With returns this high, why would a rational institution respond to Pharma's lobbying in any way other than continuing and possibly increasing this non-capital market funding? A closer review of these ratios reveals that they do not accommodate the forgone opportunities of alternative investments in health R&D (e.g, clinical trials of new service delivery models) or other ways of improving health outcomes (e.g. expanding workforce). Hence these ratios do not accommodate the full cost to society of higher prices.

The expression underlying Santerre and Vernon's estimate is generalised to the following form:

$$r = \frac{k\Delta L^{P}}{\Delta \mathcal{R}},$$

(3.1)

where k is the maxWTP for an additional year of life (and assumed to be constant regardless of the investment in R&D); ΔL^{P} is the additional life-years possible from new drugs and $\Delta \mathcal{R}$ is the additional investment in R&D, which leads to the development of additional drugs. Hence, a 28-fold return on consumers' welfare means that for every dollar of revenue from higher prices (foregone consumer welfare), the additional life-years from the additional new drugs had a monetary value of $28. This general expression is the measure of rate of return that is consistent with the prevailing political economy; the cost of increased health budget savings (reduction in $\mathcal{R}$) is decreased life-years in the future (reduction in L^{P}).

The policy narrative states (with supporting evidence) that: (1) increased R&D will lead to more drugs; and (2) drugs have an average impact on life expectancy that is greater than or equal to zero. Therefore, if prices and R&D increase, so too must the population's future health. If the policy narrative is accepted, then it is

---

[9] For countries that use CEA to inform drug reimbursement decisions, there would appear to be little value in retrospective uncontrolled studies such as these to inform pricing decisions on future drugs.

reasonable that this expression of rate of return excludes the possibility that reduced R&D will improve the population's health. However the central premise of the prevailing political economy (that the trade-off between price and future health exists) is not tested by the empirical research. Specifically, Eq. (3.1) does not accommodate the possibility that: (1) the net health effect of the drug for target patients could be positive and higher prices and hence more R&D could lead to more new drugs; but (2) the net effect of more R&D on the population's health could be negative. This finding is consistent with the observation by Comanor (1986) that the possibility that improved competition (lower prices) today and improved future health could both occur is not considered in the research agenda.

A more general expression of this return on non-capital market investment in pharmaceutical R&D would accommodate the possibility that policy can both improve competition (lower prices) and improve the population's health both today and in the future. However, before such an expression can be developed, the critical implicit assumption in the US pharma-economic literature needs to be explicated. This assumption concerns the nature (and/or the existence) of the budget constraint.

3.3 Fixed, Constrained and Unconstrained Budgets

In the simplest sense, budget constraints can be fixed, absent or something "in between". To explore the question of "in between" we need a formal distinction between the different types of budget constraints. Such a distinction is proposed by Claxton et al. (2000). In the context of a discussion about the shadow price of the budget constraint,[10] Claxton et al. raised the idea of two types of budgets for health. The magnitude of the first is defined by some decision maker external to the health sector, for example a Treasury Department official who takes into account the constraints in total government spending. This budget is set at a fixed amount and cannot be expanded. The second type of budget has a size that is defined by a decision about the maxWTP for a health effect. Any programme that meets the defined threshold can be financed, and all programmes that meet this criterion are financed. In this case, the budget expands to accommodate any programme that

---

[10] Claxton et al. (2000) distinguish between a shadow price of a budget constraint that is determined from a positive empirical question and a normative decision by a social decision maker. The exogenous shadow price is derived in a situation where the health budget is defined by a policy maker exogenous to the health care system and the shadow price of the budget constraint is defined as the marginal benefit (additional QALYs) from marginal expansion of the budget. However, when the health budget is able to be expanded, the authors argue that "there is no reason to regarding existing budgets for health care as fixed." In these cases the budget is expanded to fund all services that have a net benefit of zero or more and hence the budget can be defined as endogenous.

meets this criterion. Claxton et al. describe the latter budget as endogenous and the former as exogenous. But is this distinction between two types of budgets sufficient? The following section defines four distinct types of budgets.

3.3.1 Four Types of Budgets

In an adaption of Claxton et al., the following formal definitions of budget constraints are proposed and used throughout this book.

1. A *fixed budget* cannot be expanded and any additional purchases can be funded only if an existing activity is displaced.
2. A *constrained budget* can be expanded by a trigger such as the decision to finance a new drug but there is a foregone benefit to the expansion to finance a drug; other health and non-health programmes or investments in R&D for unpatented programmes could instead have been expanded or implemented.
3. An *unconstrained budget* is one that is expanded to accommodate any purchase that has an ICER at or below the maxWTP, where this maxWTP is defined by the social decision maker as in the endogenous budget from Claxton et al. (2000). The corollary of this definition of a budget is that there is no foregone benefit, within or external to the health sector, to any purchase with an ICER at or below that threshold. The price of a new drug is relevant to the new drug adoption decision in that the price must not be above the maxWTP.
4. *No budget* means that there is no constraint on health expenditure. The price of a new drug is not relevant to the new drug adoption decision in this context.

3.3.2 Why Is It Useful to Have Four Classifications of Budgets?

The important point about these distinctions is their implication for interpreting the benefit of new drugs. The US pharma-economic literature generally implicitly assumes that the health budget is unconstrained. In this context it is reasonable to conclude that if new drugs can be shown to have contributed to improved health of target patients in the past, then having fewer new drugs in the future will reduce the population's future health.

An example of the application of this assumption in the peer reviewed literature is Lichtenberg and Duflos (2008). The authors state that an empirical finding that 65 % of a 2-year increase in life expectancy over the period 1995–2003 can be attributed to new drugs means that if these new drugs had not been available, the increase in the life expectancy of Australians would have been 35 % of this amount, namely 0.7 years, over this period. This implicitly assumes that there is no other opportunity to improve the patient's health, other than the use of new drugs.

However, the only condition under which this claim can be made is if we assume an unconstrained budget; all other opportunities to improve health are already funded because they meet the decision threshold. Under a constrained or fixed budget, the resources allocated to the additional cost of new drugs could have otherwise been allocated to other programmes. The counterfactual to additional expenditure on new drugs would have been a world in which other services were purchased, resulting in health benefits that were either better than, less than or no different from those from the availability of more new drugs. In the context of the unconstrained budget, this counterfactual is irrelevant; if the counterfactual programme had an ICER less than or equal to the maxWTP, then it would have already been funded, and its funding would not be dependent upon the expenditure on new drugs.

Using these distinctions between types of budgets we can now prove that Santerre and Vernon's result of a 28-fold return on consumer investments via higher prices only excludes the possibility that the US could have done better with lower prices if there is an unconstrained budget. But first we start with a general expression for rate of return that accommodates all of these budgets.

3.4   Accommodating the Budget Constraint in the Return on R&D

There is more than one possible expression for a return on R&D funded by non-capital market funds, and a number will include the benefits of foregone activity, which, if it is the best alternative activity, is the opportunity cost. One general expression that accommodates the possibility that more drugs could either increase, decrease or not impact on a population's future health is presented in this section. I then show that the conventional measure of the rate of return, r [Eq. (3.1)] is a special case of the general expression, where the budget is unconstrained. Finally, I derive the conditions under which the population's future health increases if both current prices and the number of future NMEs decrease.

3.4.1   A General Expression for the Rate of Return on Consumer Investment in Pharmaceutical R&D

One general expression for return on non-capital market sourced investment in pharmaceutical R&D is:

$$e = \frac{\Delta L^P - \frac{f}{d_t}\Delta L^P}{\frac{1}{d_0}(\omega\Delta\mathcal{R} + \Delta H)},$$

(3.2)

where:

- ΔL^P is the additional health effects (L) possible from the additional new drugs (P);
- $\Delta \mathcal{R}$ is the additional investment in pharmaceutical R&D for new drugs;
- ω is the ratio of every dollar that needs to be raised by higher prices in order to finance one additional dollar of NME R&D,[11] where $3 < \omega < 5$;
- ΔH is the increased investment from the public and private not-for-profit medical research funds;
- d_i is the average incremental cost per effect of services displaced to finance the additional cost of the additional new drugs, at either the current period ($i = 0$), or the future period when the new drug is marketed, ($i = t$); and
- f is the weighted average incremental price-effectiveness ratio (IPER) of these additional new drugs.[12]

This rate of return e has four main characteristics that distinguish it from the conventional return r, as expressed in Eq. (3.1):

- The denominator captures the full financial value of the investment by the public (via higher prices and public research funders);
- The financial cost of this investment is translated into a health loss;
- The financial cost to the health budget of purchasing the new drugs is included; and
- The financial costs of the new drugs are converted to health effects.

Each of these characteristics is reviewed in detail below.

3.4.1.1   The Denominator Captures the Full Financial Value Investment

The denominator captures the full change in investment made by the non-capital market investors ($\omega\Delta\mathcal{R} + \Delta H$) and not just the resultant increase in investment by the firm ($\Delta\mathcal{R}$). This investment by the non-capital market funders comprises:

- ΔH the increase in investment from the public and private not-for-profit medical research funds, for example, the US National Institute of Health (Joint Economic Committee 2000); and
- $\omega\Delta\mathcal{R}$ the total increase in expenditure by the purchaser as a consequence of the higher prices, only a portion of which is invested into pharmaceutical R&D for new drugs according to US pharma-economists.

---

[11] The evidence for this adjustment is that around 20–30 % of the additional profit from a higher price with constant quantity purchased will be invested into R&D for new drugs hence $\frac{1}{0.3} < \omega < \frac{1}{0.2}$ (ITA 2004 p. 30).

[12] The IPER is arithmetically identical to the ICER and therefore includes adjustments to account for any net additional costs or savings elsewhere in the health system. Conceptually the IPE recognises the endogeneity of price of new drugs to the reimbursement process. Unlike the ICER of say a smoking cessation program where the only costs are the salary of a counsellor, the IPER of a drug behaves more like the price in a bilateral monopoly—it is the product of negotiation.

Why is it useful to define the investment against which the return is being assessed as the full investment by consumers via higher prices and public sector research funding ($\omega\Delta\mathcal{R} + \Delta H$), rather than $\Delta\mathcal{R}$, the changed investment by firms into R&D? The reason is that it prevents an overestimate of the return on the investment by consumers and the public sector, where this return is in the form of the number of additional new drugs in the future. In simple terms, $\Delta\mathcal{R}$ underestimates the investment required by consumers to achieve an additional drug. Therefore, by using $\Delta\mathcal{R}$ as the denominator, the return to consumer investment in overestimated. This issue is discussed in more detail in Pekarsky (2012, Appendix 7).

3.4.1.2 The Financial Cost of Investment Is Translated into a Health Loss

The financial cost of the investment ($\omega\Delta\mathcal{R} + \Delta H$) is translated to a loss in potential health benefits (a health rather than financial cost) to the population as a consequence of the services displaced to finance the additional expenditure.

In this example, this loss in health effects is derived by dividing the additional financial cost to the public sector and purchasers by d_0, the average ICER (aICER)[13] of the services displaced to finance these additional costs. This displacement occurs because the budget is assumed to be fixed. If the budget were constrained rather than fixed, the aICER of the services that could otherwise have been financed with the expanded budget would be used. Hence, the health cost to the population of higher prices and additional public sector funding of research is defined as the foregone health effects of the investment in non-capital market funded R&D, which under a fixed budget is given by the expression:

$$\frac{\omega\Delta\mathcal{R} + \Delta H}{d_0}.$$

3.4.1.3 The Financial Cost to the Health Budget of Purchasing the New Drugs Is Included

The numerator in Eq. (3.2):

$$\Delta L^P - \frac{f}{d_t}\Delta L^P,$$

accounts for the financial costs to the heath budget of additional future drugs:

---

[13] The average ICER is an average of the average.

$$f \Delta L^P.$$

New drugs are not provided free of charge by companies. It is clear to US pharma-economists that the cost to firms of manufacturing new drugs should be netted off the sales in order to estimate the rate of return to the firms of the investments in R&D. Vernon (2003) is an example of the numerous studies that examine the relationship between firm (accounting) profit as a return on pharmaceutical R&D, not firm revenue. It seems reasonable then to assume that the additional net cost to the health sector of the new drug should also be excluded from the return to the health sector from its investments in higher prices.[14]

The additional net financial cost to the health sector of the new drugs is represented by ΔC in HTA/CEA and by $f \Delta L^P$ in this ratio, where ΔL^P is the additional health effect from the new drugs and f is the weighted average IPER of these new drugs.

3.4.1.4   The Financial Costs of the New Drugs Are Converted to Health Effects

We assume, initially, that the net additional financial cost of the future new drug needs to be financed from within a fixed budget. Services need to be displaced in order to finance the additional financial cost to the health sector of adopting the future new drug. The aICER of the displaced services in the future (time $= t$) are given by d_t. Hence, the numerator, ΔL, the net effect of more R&D today on the population's future health, is:

$$\Delta L = \Delta L^P - \frac{f}{d_t} \Delta L^P.$$

This represents the health gain to the target patients for the new drug, ΔL^P, less ΔL^D the loss in health to other patients in the population due to the financing the additional cost of the future new drugs by displacing programmes with an aICER of d, where:

$$\Delta L^D = \frac{f \Delta L^P}{d_t}.$$

---

[14] The question of whether the economic rent to the firm should be included in the estimate of the impact of new drug R&D is discussed in detail in Chap. 10. In this chapter the question is: what is the return to the consumer of their investment in new Drug R&D via higher prices?

Assume for simplicity that the cost per effect of displaced services is constant over time:

$$d = d_0 = d_t.$$

Then Eq. (3.2) is rearranged to provide an estimate of the return on the non-capital market investment:

$$e = \frac{\Delta L^P (d - f)}{(\omega \Delta \mathcal{R} + \Delta H)}. \qquad (3.3)$$

This equation is saying that the return on consumers' and the public sectors' full investment into more future drugs is the additional health effects from that drug with a monetary value given by the difference between the ICER of the health effects displaced and the IPER of the health effects from new drugs. The drivers of the return e include four parameters not identified in the conventional measure of return, r. These parameters are: d, f, ω, and ΔH. The aICER of displaced services, d is relevant because it signals the health value of the additional resources used to finance higher prices. The higher the aICER of displaced services, the less health effects can be purchased from the additional savings available to consumers with lower prices. The IPER of the new drug f, is relevant because the higher it is, the higher the additional costs of the future new drugs and the more health effects need to be displaced (health programmes contracted) to finance the new drugs. The proportion of additional funds raised by higher prices that is invested in NME R&D (ω) is relevant because the higher this proportion is, the greater the number of future NMEs per dollar of higher prices today. Finally, it is not only higher prices that finance pharmaceutical R&D. A significant share is financed by health research institutes, both private-not-for-profit and public (ΔH).

Unlike the conventional US estimate r, e is not a function of the choice of the maxWTP, k. This situation is a consequence of converting the financial costs of additional financial expenditure today and in the future, into foregone health effects.

In summary, this alternative rate of return captures the net effect on the population's health of the non-capital market funded investment in increased R&D by firms.

The general expression presented in this section is one of a number of possible options. Other possible expressions include using an opportunity cost rather than a simple net population benefit. (See Chaps. 6 and 7)

Now we compare Eq. (3.1)

$$r = \frac{k \Delta L^P}{\Delta \mathcal{R}},$$

and Eq. (3.3)

$$e = \frac{\Delta L^P (d - f)}{(\omega \Delta \mathcal{R} + \Delta H)}.$$

This comparison illustrates why r is a special case of e. The former assumes that there are no health effects foregone in order to achieve the additional benefits of the new drugs, either in terms of higher prices today or higher expenditure on more drugs tomorrow. While this situation ($d = 0$, $\omega = 1$, $\Delta H = 0$) could apply in the US, at least in the minds of decision makers and consumers (Weinstein 2008), it is unlikely to apply in other countries throughout the OECD and it certainly does not apply in the country in which the Reimburser makes decisions. It is a special, rather than a general, case.

We now address this situation formally.

3.5   Conditions Under Which More Future NMEs Means Less Future Health

Now we return to the central premise of the prevailing political economy: the increased health of the population is positively related to the number of additional NMEs in the future and hence positively related to higher prices today. Is it possible for there to be a net increase in the future health of the population as a consequence of reduced investments by the non-capital market sources, even if the conventionally measured return on this investment is estimated to be 28:1?

The net effect on the population's future health of more new drugs in the future is given by the numerator of Eq. (3.2):

$$\Delta L = \Delta L^P - \frac{f}{d} \Delta L^P.$$

That is, the net health gain to the population is the health gain from the additional drugs less the health gain from what is displaced to finance the additional cost of the new drug.

If the net effect on the future population is negative (there is less health as a consequence of more future new drugs) then:

$$\Delta L = d \Delta L^P - f \Delta L^P < 0,$$

where $\Delta L^P, d > 0$

$$\Rightarrow d - f < 0$$
$$\Rightarrow 0 < d < f. \tag{3.4}$$

This result simply says that if the aICER of the services displaced to finance the new drug is less than the IPER of the new drug, then the effect of purchasing the additional new drug in the future is a net reduction in the population's health. The conventional rate of return,

$$r = \frac{k\Delta L^P}{\mathcal{R}},$$

is constant regardless of the relationship between d and f. It is also constant regardless of the price, f, of the new drug. Therefore it is possible that $r \gg 1$ even though there is a net reduction in the population's health. That is, $r > 1$ is not a sufficient condition to ensure that there will be a net gain in the population's health.

Is the condition $d < f$ plausible? That is, is it possible that the aICER of the services that are displaced are lower than the aICER of the health effects of the new drug? It is plausible in the context of a decision to adopt a specific new drug when budgets are fixed. An example of how this situation could arise is the case of health budgets across the UK being required by law to purchase the breast cancer drug trastuzumab for eligible patients because it was established by the National Institute for Health Clinical Excellence (NICE) as being a "cost-effective" drug. The significant additional financial costs of trastuzumab needed to be financed by displacing other cancer drugs and therapies for which there was no legal require-ment for them to be reimbursed by the funder. If these other programmes were more cost-effective than the new drug, then the net effect would have been a reduction in the health of the population (Barrett et al. 2006). It is also possible that the role of institutions such as NICE and Pharmaceutical Benefit Advisory Committee (PBAC), in providing incentives for evidence development for patented inputs without addressing the failure of the market to develop evidence of unpatented inputs, have increased the probability that $d < f$.[15]

---

[15] Significantly, institutions such as NICE, PBAC and the Australian Medical Services Advisory Committee (MSAC) with their preference for financing programmes and technologies that have demonstrated cost-effectiveness could be increasing the probability that $d < f$.

First, the availability of evidence of cost and effect is biased towards programs for which the market and institutions provide incentives for an evidence base. A focus on HTA/CEA generated evidence to inform decisions can be justified as consistent with Evidence Based Medicine (EBM). However, EBM does not recognise the failure of markets and institutions to provide incentives for the development of evidence for non-patented or unpatentable technologies. Hence, it is likely that there are programs that are cost-effective, but are not funded because the market has failed to provide incentives to develop evidence of cost and effect.

Second, the process of displacement to finance new drugs is biased towards programs that have not been approved as part of formal evidence based reimbursement process. If a program is recommended or reimbursed via an EBM decision process, then the capacity of the system to displace this program in order to access the funds for a newly reimbursed service is limited. This is particularly relevant if there is a financial incentive to prevent this displacement (a patent for example). Additionally, a program for which there is no evidence of cost and effect can be displaced more easily than one for which there is evidence of "cost-effectiveness".

Therefore, to the extent that increased probability of being displaced is correlated with less available evidence rather than the underlying cost-effectiveness of the program, it is feasible that there are situations where $d < f$ and hence the net effect of reimbursement on a population is

It can be concluded that, if the health budget is unconstrained, a positive relationship between more NMEs and more population health can be deduced from the result of the conventional rate of return (*e*) of around 28-fold. In this case there is no health loss to either the additional costs of R&D or the additional costs of the future drug hence the entire benefit of the additional drugs is appropriated as additional health effects. However, if the budget is fixed rather than unconstrained this assumed relationship, and hence the central premise of the current political economy, is an empirical question. The direction of the net effect of more NMEs on the population health depends upon the relationship between the IPERs for the new drug and aICERs of the displaced services. In turn this relationship depends upon a range of institutional and market arrangements and incentives, particularly the differential impacts of incentives and reimbursement decisions on patented versus unpatented technologies and programmes.

What about the case of the constrained budget where services do not need to be physically displaced and the budget can be expanded, but there are competing uses of the expanded budget?

3.6   The Conventional Rate of Return and the Constrained Budget

What are the conditions under which lower prices in the past for drugs and less drugs today could have led to better health today, if budgets are constrained (rather than fixed or unconstrained)? The possibility for better health today if prices were lower is discussed in this section in the context of the US rather than another country, for three reasons. The first reason is that the US is the only country for which there is an estimate of a return on increased price of new drugs. Second, the possibility that the US could have done better had it not maintained higher drug prices and instead invested in other technologies or improved access to all health care is not even considered as a possibility in the prevailing PEND in the US. Third, relative to other countries such as Australia, Canada and UK, the US budget is constrained rather fixed. From 1990 to 2010 the US had the greatest increases in the percentage of the GDP that is expended on either health or pharmaceuticals.[16] However, the US health budget is not unconstrained. If the health budgets were unconstrained, the US could have had both higher prices to the producer today and subsidised the price of drugs to consumers (improved access), both of which would have represented an additional cost to the US health budgets. Essentially, the idea of the trade-off between savings (or improved access) today and health tomorrow,

---

negative. Furthermore, the greater the bias in funding technologies for which there is no failure in the market for evidence, the greater the probability that $d < f$.

[16] See Pekarsky (2012, Appendix 3).

which is a central theme of the US policy narrative, would not be relevant in a society that had an unconstrained health budget.[17]

3.6.1   The Conditions Under Which Fewer Future NMEs and More Future Health Is Possible

The following condition in a constrained budget would lead to the possibility that at lower prices and with fewer additional NMEs in the past years, the population's health could be better off today, despite having received less additional health effects from new pharmaceuticals:

- The availability of an alternative option to the investment of $\omega\Delta\mathcal{R}$ in new drug R&D, for example the extension of an existing programme or an unpatented medical innovation, where the resultant health effects have a lower cost per effect compared to those of the new drugs.

Consider the case of a constrained budget; it can be expanded to accommodate the additional financial costs of the new drug, but as a consequence of this expansion the benefits of other services that could also have been adopted are forgone. In this situation the net impact on the health of the population is the same as the effect for the target patients. Furthermore, it is reasonable to assume that the expected net effect of adopting a new drug for a patient group is positive because the drug regulation process is intended to minimise the risk of a net negative effect on patients' health from new drugs, even though some authors argue that this regulation in fact unnecessarily delays new drug approvals (Philipson et al. 2008; Vernon et al. 2009).

However, if the counterfactual to purchasing new drugs with additional funds were a more cost-effective strategy, then there is a net economic loss from the strategy of investing in more future NMEs, even if there is a net increase in population health from NMEs. Furthermore, alternative historic investments in R&D in technologies other than new drugs could have resulted in more cost-effective new technologies. In short, it is possible that a country such as the US could be better off today had it had lower drug prices in the past, if it had a constrained budget and/or options other than additional expenditure on new drugs to improve health.

This result (lower prices in the past, fewer drugs today and more health today) is possible, even if the estimate that there is a 28:1 return from investment in pharmaceutical R&D via higher prices is accurate, for at least two reasons. First, the return in terms of additional possible health effects from alternative investments could be the same as for new drugs, but the return to consumers could be higher,

---

[17] The US pharma-economic literature is not consistent in this position. Some of the US pharma-economic analysis implicitly assumes that the budget is unconstrained.

simply because the price per future health effect is lower. Second, the costs of achieving a given innovative health effect could have been much lower, simply because the associated investment is lower.

This result simply reinforces a fundamental principle of economics, opportunity cost. If we are selecting the strategy that maximises health, then this is also the selection that minimises the opportunity cost. If the opportunity cost of the action is greater than the benefit of the action then the population would have been better off by funding that alternative action instead.

However, the point remains that the US has had a dramatic 10 year increase in longevity since 1960 and retrospective analyses seem to suggest that much of this health gain can be explained by the availability of new drugs. Given this evidence, is it plausible that the US, with its focus on rapid uptake of new technologies, could have done better with lower drug prices and fewer new drugs?[18]

3.6.2   Is It Plausible That the Counterfactual World Could Have Been Healthier?

If the evidence of the aICER of the counterfactual programmes could be compared with the IPER of new drugs, then it would be possible to test empirically this question of whether the US could have done better with lower prices. Unfortunately, as is the case with much of the rest of the OECD, there is comparatively less evidence on the counterfactual to increased expenditure on patented technologies for example, unpatented respite care programmes. The reasons for this include the failure of the market to provide evidence of unpatented programs and the failure of institutions to address this market failure. This point is a major theme throughout this book.

In the absence of evidence of the counterfactual to historic drug expenditure in the US, there is an alternative option available to assess the question. When we look at the evidence beyond the US, the possibility that its population could have done better becomes apparent. The absence of evidence of the counterfactual in the US is no longer a barrier to determining whether it is reasonable to exclude the possibility that the US could have done better with lower drug prices and fewer NMEs. This evidence is discussed in detail in and Pekarsky (2012, Appendix 3).

In summary, at 10 years, the increase in longevity experienced by the US over the period 1960–2008 could be significant (PhRMA 2011), however, this literature does not refer to the increase in average longevity of the US population relative to the rest of the OECD. For any two points in time during the period 1960–2008, the longevity of the US population increased by less than that of countries such as Australia, Canada and the UK. This difference is not insignificant. In 2009, the life

---

[18] A number of studies have shown that the US has shorter delay times for new drug adoption (Danzon et al. 2005).

expectancy at birth was estimated at 80 years for an Australian male, compared with 76 years for a US male, a difference that is equivalent to 40 % of the growth in life expectancy in the US over the 48 years to 2008 (Pekarsky (2012, Appendix 3). This represented an improvement of 6 and 4 years in life expectancy since 1990 for an Australian and a US male, respectively. Hence the gain in average life expectancy at birth for a US citizen was only two thirds of the gain for an Australian citizen.

This evidence is not sufficient to prove that the US could have done better had they lowered prices and instead invested in other health programmes, in health workforce and improved access to health care for the uninsured. It simply identifies the evidence missing from the current US policy narrative. This evidence could convince decision makers that, while new drugs could have contributed to 60 % of the 10 years of growth in life expectancy in the US, this does not mean even more drugs are essential to achieve continuing improvements in life expectancy. Perhaps looking beyond the US to consider the options taken by other countries should be part of the US policy choice set.

From the perspective of this book and its focus on the PEND, the omission of the evidence of the US life expectancy gains relative to those in the rest of the OECD from the US policy narrative is significant. The omission excludes consideration of the possibility the US could have achieved more with lower drug prices and more expenditure on other areas, including improved access to new drugs. Had US Pharma introduced this issue into the policy narrative, they would have had to consider the possibility that the health of the US population could have been better than it is today, despite the significant increases over the previous 50 years.

3.7 Discussion and Conclusions

3.7.1 The Reimburser's Question

The Reimburser reviews her question.

- Does the US estimate of a 28-fold health return on pharmaceutical R&D financed by higher drug prices exclude the possibility that at lower prices and with fewer NMEs the US population's longevity would now be even higher?

The gain in average life expectancy at birth in the US since 1960 and the contribution of new drugs to this is an important theme in the US policy narrative. The evidence that there is a 28:1 return could have some influence in the US as part of the strategy to lobby to maintain higher prices. This evidence is not sufficient to persuade the rest of the OECD that increased prices will lead to better outcomes for these countries. One reason is that this result does not exclude the possibility that if US health budget holders had made other investments in the past, health today would have been better. Furthermore, it is not just the estimate of return on pharmaceutical R&D derived using Eq. (3.1) that excludes the possibility that the US was worse off with higher prices: the prevailing PEND excludes the possibility of increased prices today and worse health tomorrow. The omission of the evidence of the US life expectancy gains relative to the rest of the OECD from the US policy narrative is a significant advantage to the prevailing US policy narrative. It means that pharma-economists do not need to explain whether the US could have achieved more with lower drug prices and more expenditure on other areas, including improved access to current drugs through more subsidies. In simple terms, the prevailing PEND can accommodate variation in the size of the costs compared with the benefits of lower drug prices $(0 < r < 200)$, but it cannot accommodate the possibility that higher prices leads to less health, that is, $r < 0$.

3.7.2 Conclusion

The Reimburser reflects on the situation. Twenty years of application of economic evaluation and a decision threshold to new drug reimbursement decisions has improved the information available to the new drug reimbursement process.

The use of economic evaluation has also improved the confidence with which a government can defend a decision to finance a new high-cost drug; it might have a significant additional financial cost to the drug budget, but at least it is "value for money".[19] But did the strategy of a threshold price for new drugs result in reimbursement decisions that increased the population's health? Or were the programmes displaced to finance these new drugs more cost-effective than the new drugs? Did this strategy of using HTA/CEA ensure that the best use was made of the entire health budget? Or did it create a system in which programmes that were unpatented or unpatentable could not access or compete against because there was a failure of the market to provide evidence of their cost and effect? Did the institution's attempts to correct the failure of the free market to generate evidence of the incremental cost and effect of new drugs generate other problems? In the words of Arrow (1963):

> The social adjustment towards optimality thus puts obstacles in its own path. (p. 947)

The Reimburser is concerned that she has a long journey ahead to answer the Ministers' question: How should she respond to the claim that a decision threshold that is below the FPP is worse for the population? She is clear of the next step; an understanding of exactly what Pharma is claiming there will be less of if new drug prices are lower. The value of the desired outcome of R&D—clinical innovation—is the subject of the next chapter.

---

[19] The Health Minister said this to the Reimburser after she approved a very high cost drug with a significant additional cost to the health budget. The Health Minister expressed his relief at being able to provide Treasury with a "solid economic rationale" for this unexpected increase in the drug budget, namely that it was "cost-effective" and "value for money".

References

Arrow KJ (1963) Uncertainty and the welfare economics of medical care. Am Econ Rev LIII (5):941–972

Barrett A, Riques T, Small M, Smith R (2006) How much will Herceptin really cost? Br Med J 333:1118–1120

Claxton K, Lacey LF, Walker SG (2000) Selecting treatments: a decision theoretic approach. J R Stat Soc 163(2):211–225

Comanor WS (1986) The political economy of the pharmaceutical industry. J Econ Lit 24 (3):1178–1217

Cremieux P, Jarninen D, Long G, Merrigan P (2007) Pharmaceutical spending and health outcomes. In: Sloan F, Hsieh C-R (eds) Pharmaceutical innovation: incentives, competition, and cost-benefit analysis in international perspective. Cambridge University Press, New York, pp 226–241

Danzon PM, Wang YR, Wang L (2005) The impact of price regulation on the launch delay of new drugs—evidence from twenty-five major markets in the 1990s. Health Econ 14(3):269–292. doi:10.1002/hec.931

DiMasi JA, Hansen RW, Grabowski HG (2003) The price of innovation: new estimates of drug development costs. J Health Econ 22(2):151–185

Giaccotto C, Santerre RE, Vernon JA (2005) Drug prices and research and development investment behavior in the pharmaceutical industry. J Law Econ 48(1):195–214

Golec J, Hegde S, Vernon J (2005) Pharmaceutical R&D spending and threats of price regulation. J Financ Quant Anal 45(1):239–264

International Trade Administration (2004) Pharmaceutical price controls in OECD countries: implications for U.S. consumers, pricing, research and development, and innovation. US Department of Commerce, Washington, DC

Joint Economic Committee (2000) The benefits of medical research and the role of the NIH. GPO, Washington, DC

Lichtenberg FR (2004) Sources of U.S. longevity increase, 1960-2001. Q Rev Econ Finance 44 (3):369–389

Lichtenberg FR, Duflos G (2008) Pharmaceutical innovation and the longevity of Australians: a first look. National Bureau of Economic Research, Inc, NBER Working Papers: 14009

Pekarsky BAK (2012) Trust, constraints and the counterfactual: reframing the political economy of new drug price. Dissertation, University of Adelaide, http://digital.library.adelaide.edu.au/dspace/handle/2440/79171. Accessed 25 Dec 2013

Philipson TJ, Berndt ER, Gottschalk AHB, Sun EC (2008) Cost-benefit analysis of the FDA: the case of the Prescription Drug User Fee Acts. J Public Econ 92(5–6):1306–1325

PhRMA (2011) Access and Affordability. Pharmaceutical Research and Manufacturers of America. http://www.phrma.org/issues/access-affordability. Accessed 19 May 2011

Santerre RE, Vernon JA (2006) Assessing consumer gains from a drug price control policy in the United States. South Econ J 73(1):233–245

Sloan FA, Hsieh C-R (2007) Conclusions and policy implications. In: Sloan FA, Ruey HC (eds) Pharmaceutical innovation: incentives, competition, and cost-benefit analysis in international perspective. Cambridge University Press, New York, pp 262–277

Vernon JA (2003) The relationship between price regulation and pharmaceutical profit margins. Appl Econ Lett 10(8):467–470

Vernon JA (2004) Pharmaceutical R&D investment and cash flows: an instrumental variables approach to testing for capital market imperfections. J Pharm Finance Econ Policy 13(4):3–17

Vernon JA, Golec JH, Lutter R, Nardinelli C (2009) An exploratory study of FDA new drug review times, Prescription Drug User Fee Acts, and R&D spending. Q Rev Econ Finance 49(4):1260–1274

Weinstein MC (2008) How much are Americans willing to pay for a quality-adjusted life year? Med Care 46(4):343–345

Wu SY, Lindgren B (1984) Social and private rates of returns derived from pharmaceutical innovations: some empirical findings. In: Pharmaceutical economics: papers presented at the 6th Arne Ryde symposium, Helsingborg, Sweden 1982. Malmo, Sweden: Liber, pp 217–254

Chapter 4
The Clinical Value of Innovation

Abstract The term "innovation" is used in a number of different ways in pharmaceutical regulation processes. In this chapter I address the question of what is meant by the term "innovation" in the context of the debate on new drug prices. I distinguish between lay and medical uses of the terms "innovation" and "innovative" then I identify three ways that pharmaceutical innovation generates a social surplus. First, clinical innovation, which is the "incremental effect" used in cost-effectiveness analysis and quantified for a specific clinical context and patient group. Resource innovation is the second source of surplus: innovation in the resources involved in supplying a given clinical benefit, for example, an oral version of an intravenous drug. Third, developing and manufacturing innovation, for example, innovation in the methods of manufacturing drugs. An analogy between clinical and economic concepts of value is noted. Clinical value of innovation, like economic value, is constrained by the best alternative strategy. The clinical value of a new drug's innovation is its gross clinical effect (compared with no care) constrained by the opportunity cost (foregone health benefit) to the patient of not using the best existing therapy.

4.1 The Reimburser's Problem

The US International Trade Delegate is arguing that pharmaceutical regulation needs to "reward innovation" and that the pricing system in the country of interest does not achieve this. The Reimburser is aware that a recent decision about a new drug was controversial because the Reimburser refused to pay more for that drug (on a cost per course basis) compared with a drug that had been off-patent for at least 5 years (a generic). The reason for her decision was that the new drug was shown in clinical trials to be no more effective than the existing generic drug. The new drug was innovative in that it had a different molecular structure from any existing drug, and it was even the lead drug in a new therapeutic sub-class[1];

---

[1] An example of a new therapeutic subclass is the introduction of the selective serotonin reuptake inhibitors (SSRIs) in the early 1990s. SSRIs are anti-depressants that were considered a separate

© Springer International Publishing Switzerland 2015

B.A.K. Pekarsky, *The New Drug Reimbursement Game*,

DOI 10.1007/978-3-319-08903-4_4

however, the new drug did not provide a clinical advantage over the standard therapy for this condition. The International Trade Delegate argues that a significant investment was made into researching and developing this innovative drug and the higher price was needed to reward this investment in innovation. The International Trade Delegate points out that the firm that took this risk and invested would have been better off if it had simply produced the generic. Where is the incentive for innovative firms to take risks if they are rewarded no more than generic firms that take no risks? He argues that it does not make economic sense for this investment in the innovation process to remain unrewarded.

The Reimburser is concerned about the concepts of innovation revealed by the discussion with the US International Trade Delegate. From a clinical perspective, the value of innovation is about the clinical benefit of the new drug, not about the characteristics of the molecule or the type of risks taken by the firm. However, the Health Economic Adviser points out that clinical innovation is not necessary for there to be pharmaceutical innovation. A new drug could be no more effective than an existing drug but delivered in a way that does not require a hospital admission, hence reducing the cost associated with administering the drug. Hence the innovation in this case is not about clinical benefit; it is about resource benefit.

Is there a fundamental difference between how economists and clinicians understand the value of pharmaceutical innovation? The Reimburser asks her Health Economic Adviser:

- Is there a way of defining the value of pharmaceutical innovation that makes sense from both an economic and clinical perspective?

4.2   Innovation: Lay, Regulatory and Medical Concepts

4.2.1   Innovation and the Regulatory Process

The term "innovative" is used to distinguish between generic firms (that do not invest in pharmaceutical R&D and only produce generic drugs) and innovative firms (that do invest in pharmaceutical R&D).[2] If an innovative firm develops a new

---

therapeutic subclass from the existing tricyclic anti-depressants (TCAs). Fluoxetine was the first SSRI (innovative) and then others ("me-toos") followed (e.g. sertraline). The introduction of venlafaxine in the late 1990s was considered to be a new therapeutic subclass, the serotonin–norepinephrine reuptake inhibitors (SNRIs) (DeVane 1994; Pekarsky 2010).

[2] This characteristic of a firm, investment in pharmaceutical R&D, is a necessary condition for membership in the PhRMA: "The Pharmaceutical Manufacturers Association was founded in 1958." Its name was changed to the Pharmaceutical Research and Manufacturers of America in 1994 to underscore the extraordinary commitment of member companies to research. Headquartered in Washington, DC, PhRMA represents the country's leading pharmaceutical research and biotechnology companies, which are "devoted to inventing medicines that allow patients to live longer, healthier and more productive lives" (PhRMA 2013).

molecule, it only needs to establish a sufficient degree of physical difference from an existing technology to be defined as an "innovation" or "invention". For example, a New Molecular Entity (NME) can be awarded a patent provided it is different from any existing molecule. Whether it is more or less effective than a placebo is not relevant to the decision to define it as "innovative" or an "invention" for the purpose of a patent. Consequently, each year there are many more molecules patented and tested in phase 1 trials than there are NMEs registered by the FDA (approved for therapeutic use).[3, 4]

For a firm to be provided with a licence to market that drug, it requires evidence of the clinical value of this innovative molecule, typically evidence of its safety and efficacy.[5] In most jurisdictions, the minimum evidence of clinical value of innovation is obtained by controlling (constraining) the effect of the new drug by some alternative therapy. For the firm to obtain a licence to market a new drug in the US it requires evidence of its performance against placebo, preferably derived from a double-blind randomised controlled trial (RCT). The evidentiary and performance demands on a licenced drug (one that is approved by an agency such as the FDA in addition to being patented) are therefore much higher than those on an innovative molecule (one that is awarded a patent). Some new drugs that are approved by the FDA are referred to as "innovative" to distinguish between first-in-class (innovative or lead) and follow-on ("me-too") drugs (Pekarsky 2010). However, not all drugs that are approved for use or described as "innovative" necessarily have a clinical value in the underlying innovation. So what is clinical innovation?

4.2.2 Clinical Innovation

HTA/CEA informs the so-called "fourth hurdle" of regulation where the quantification of the new drug's clinical innovation is the primary objective of the analysis.[6] The regulatory imperative of reimbursement decisions is to assess the appropriateness of changed, additional or substituted therapy. Therefore, reimbursing institutions are interested in the clinical value of innovation for a group of patients for whom a subsidy for the cost of the drug is being proposed. A common definition of the clinical value of innovation of a new technology is the best

---

[3] For example, in 2011 Pfizer reported 93 NMEs in the pipeline of which 4 were in the Registration phase and 13, 28 and 49 of which were in Phase 3, 2, and 1 respectively. It is not possible to determine the number of NMEs with Pfizer patents on this date, but not yet in Phase 1, from this report.

[4] A search of the Australian patent data base on February 28 2011 of patents where the applicant's name contains the word Pfizer contains 2,513 results, not all of which are NMEs (AUSPAT 2011).

[5] The US Food and Drug Administration website details the requirements for approval (FDA 2013).

[6] A paper by Cohen et al. (2007) describes the fourth hurdle and also describes some of the limitations of not considering the opportunity costs of decisions.

estimate of the additional clinical effect (or effects) of the new technology compared to the best existing therapy for the group of patients for whom its use is being assessed.[7,8] This definition requires specificity in the assessment of the "clinical value of innovation" of a new technology. For example, an HTA/CEA assessor is unlikely to ask the question: "Is this new drug clinically innovative?" Instead he might ask: "If current best therapy is replaced by this new drug for this patient group, using this clinical protocol (tests, dose and duration of therapy) what is the expected incremental effect as measured by this set of clinical endpoints?"

HTA/CEA typically involves meta-analyses of the evidence of effect from RCTs and the extrapolation of this evidence to longer time periods, additional patient groups and clinical endpoints by way of pharmaco-economic models. Uncertainty is characterised and analysed using deterministic and probabilistic sensitivity analyses. The net financial implication to the health budget of adoption, ΔC, is also estimated. (See the discussion about resource innovation in Sect. 4.3.) The incremental financial cost, ΔC, and incremental effect, ΔE, of the new drug compared with the best alternative therapy are summarised as either an incremental cost-effectiveness ratio:

$$ \text{ICER} = \frac{\Delta C}{\Delta E}, $$

or a net benefit (NB) metric:

$$ \text{NB}_i = i\Delta E - \Delta C, $$

[7] In 1993, the Australian PBAC published the first Guidelines for the use of HTA/CEA to inform a drug reimbursement process. These Guidelines illustrate the rigour and specificity HTA/CEA requires for Industry submissions to PBAC for reimbursement of new drugs. This set of guidelines is regularly updated (PBAC 2013).

[8] The US has only recently started to consider the idea of comparative effectiveness as a way of understanding the benefits of a new drug. In recent years the US has focused on evidence of performance against placebo rather than an alternative active therapy as an indicator of the value of a new drug. In the words of the FDA: "FDA's experience with comparative effectiveness claims is relatively limited. Our enabling law (FDC Act, as amended in 1962) does not require assessment of comparative assessment and the legislative history made it very clear that there is no relative effectiveness requirement. A new drug does not have to be better than or even as good as existing treatment" (Temple 2010). This statement suggests that the US decision makers conflate the idea of having to be proven to be more effective than existing therapies in order to be approved by the FDA and having to provide evidence of comparative effectiveness as part of the new drug approval for uptake on the formularies. Comparative effectiveness analysis also concerns the review of data bases such as cancer registries and longitudinal data bases held by Medicare and Medicaid to develop evidence of comparative effectiveness. The substantial infrastructure investment by the US in relation to data collection for comparative effectiveness is reviewed in Trontell (2010).

where i is some monetary value of the clinical effect.[9] [See Pekarsky (2012, Appendix 4) for a discussion of this terminology.]

This information is then used in conjunction with a range of other evidence to inform the decision to reimburse that drug.[10] While HTA/CEA methods vary across jurisdictions, there is a key common element; the focus on the estimate of ΔE for a specific clinical context (comparator, patient group and clinical protocol). A drug might be described generally as clinically innovative, but the estimate of value of clinical innovation is specific to a clinical context.

4.3 Non-clinical Pharmaceutical Innovation

The focus on clinical innovation (ΔE) as the tangible (and valuable) outcome of pharmaceutical innovation is consistent with the narrative around medical research more generally: it is about developing cures and treatment for diseases and improving life expectancy and quality of life for patients.[11] However, pharmaceutical innovation (the product of pharmaceutical R&D) can take at least two other forms and still potentially impact on population health, without having any clinical innovation content in the new drug. The first form is in relation to the implications for health resource use generally and the second relates to innovation in the drug manufacturing process.

4.3.1 Resource Innovation

The incremental impact of a new drug on resource use is:

- The conventional ΔC (the net financial impact of adopting the new drug compared to existing therapy);
- Less the share of that additional financial cost that is attributed to either:

  - The financial cost of the new drug less the financial cost of the drug that it substitutes for; or
  - The financial cost of the new drug if it is added to existing therapy (no substitution).

---

[9] The ICER does not appropriately accommodate the situation where either or both of the incremental cost and effect are negative. Hence the NB_i is considered preferable. However, in this book the situation of interest is where there is both an additional cost and an additional effect.

[10] The references and guides for pharmaco-economics and HTA/CEA are extensive. The following three articles are examples of the contributions made by economists to the HTA/CEA process (O'Brien 1996; Briggs and O'Brien 2001; Briggs et al. 2002).

[11] The American Pharmaceutical Research and Manufacturer's Association website is rich in examples of this narrative, for example, the marketing publication entitled: "2011s New Medicines Fought Wide Range of Diseases, Conditions" (PhRMA 2011).

We start with an example of pure resource innovation: a new formulation of a drug that allows the drug to be taken orally at home rather than intravenously as part of a hospital admission. This innovation could result in a reduction in the non-drug costs of \$250 per course of the drug. In this case, the difference in resource use is captured in the ICER or NBi via ΔC. From an economic perspective, this innovation can be valued in terms of increased population health, for example if the additional financial savings are allocated to other health services. However, if the firm prices the new drug so as the additional savings are entirely offset by the additional cost of the drug, then the entire value of the resource innovation is appropriated by the firm.[12] For this reason, ΔC only captures "resource innovation" if the net additional cost of the new drug relative to the existing substituted drug is excluded.[13, 14]

4.3.2   Manufacturing Innovation

Another form of non-clinical innovation is in the manufacturing process. Typically the variable costs of producing drugs is argued to be low relative to the cost of R&D; however, there remains scope to reduce the manufacturing costs.[15,16] Reduced cost of manufacturing is the source of innovation used by Tirole (1988) to illustrate the "pure value of innovation." Tirole shows how if the firm is a

---

[12] The endogeneity of new drug price is discussed further in Chap. 6.

[13] Why should the resource innovation be considered in terms of the incremental cost net the effect of the incremental cost of the drug itself? The incremental cost includes a term relating to the net financial effect of adoption on other resources, as well as the additional cost of the new drug compared to the existing drug (if it is a direct substitution.) However, as first discussed in Chap. 6, while differences in resource use and the associated costs can be estimated empirically in a clinical trial, the price of the drug and its associated cost is determined endogenously to the Reimbursement process. What this means is that a new drug could be innovative in terms of preventing the need for an admission to deliver the drug IV, however, the incremental cost will not reflect this if the firm prices the drug so as to appropriate the full value of that surplus or resource innovation. That the price of the new drug is the mechanism by which clinical and resource innovation are appropriated by the firm, a point well understood by pharma-economists, for example Vernon et al. (2009).

[14] Technically we could consider an incremental cost as resource innovation (albeit undesirable)— for example, two additional consultations with a GP are required.

[15] DiMasi's study (2002) highlighted a range of factors that could be addressed to improve productivity of drug development processes, including both regulatory and business decision making. He concluded that there could be a "substantial" impact on R&D costs if efficiency of manufacturer and research wee improved.

[16] There are numerous businesses offering innovative solutions to pharmaceutical manufacturers to improve their efficiency. A quick look at an industry journal such as the Pharmaceutical Manufacturing magazine highlights that pharmaceutical manufacturers are like every other industry—they welcome innovation in the manufacturing process (Pharmaceutical Manufacturing 2013).

monopolist in its output market it can maintain a price per unit of the good following innovation in manufacturing and the entire surplus is appropriated by the firm. In more competitive situations financial savings will be shared with purchasers. This example of innovation in manufacturing is expanded in Chap. 10 in terms of its implications for the pricing of drugs today in order to gain innovation in the future.

4.4 Discussion and Conclusion

4.4.1 What Did the AUSFTA Conclude?

The confusion in the US between innovative drugs and clinically innovative drugs could be a consequence of the US imperative to distinguish between the generic and the innovative sectors of the pharmaceutical industry; the latter does need to invest in pharmaceutical R&D whereas the former does not. However, the prevailing PEND is unequivocal: the primary value of pharmaceutical R&D is in its impact on a population's health; the ability to cure and treat disease and improve or extend quality of life [Chap. 1 and see Pekarsky (2012, Appendix 2)].

Despite the confusion in the US Congress and Senate about the distinction between innovative drugs (non-generic drugs) and clinically innovative drugs, the AUSFTA ultimately made this distinction. From Annex-2-C-Pharmaceuticals comes the following statement:

> (d) the need to recognize the value of innovative pharmaceuticals through the operation of competitive markets or by adopting or maintaining procedures that appropriately value the objectively demonstrated therapeutic significance of a pharmaceutical. (DFAT 2009)

In other words, according to the AUSFTA, the value of innovative drugs is derived from their therapeutic significance, not simply from the fact that they are molecularly distinct drugs that are the result of investment in pharmaceutical R&D. Given the significance of clinical innovation in the PEND, this outcome might come as no surprise.

4.4.2 Other Results of Pharmaceutical Innovation

The identification of three aspects of pharmaceutical innovation, all of which are products of pharmaceutical R&D, is a reminder that the economic concept of pharmaceutical innovation is broader than the pure clinical concept. Clinical and resource innovations are consistent with the policy narrative about the benefits of investing in more drugs; the advantages are not just more health but also more medical savings (Giaccotto et al. 2005).

The idea that new drugs generate savings is an increasingly important part of the global policy narrative. Personalised medicine is a current example of the imperative for resource innovation. Advocates of targeting by pharmacogenomic markers highlight the promise of innovation leading to improved sustainability of the health care sector (Davis et al. 2009; Personalized Medicine Coalition 2010). Innovation in manufacturing is a source of improved profitability for firms. One of the limitations of HTA/CEA is that while it isolates clinical innovation, ΔE, it does not isolate the resource innovation (this is integrated with the price of the new drug in ΔC) and completely ignores manufacturing innovation. Pharmacogenomics is also argued to contribute to manufacturing innovation (Cook et al. 2009).

4.4.3   Opportunity Cost and Clinical Value of Innovation

The methods developed in HTA/CEA have important implications for how we understand the process of quantifying the "objectively demonstrated therapeutic significance of a pharmaceutical". These methods highlight that if the Reimburser wants to assess the decision whether or not to replace an existing technology with a new innovative technology, she needs to define the clinical value of innovation of an NME in terms of specific clinical context. Characteristics that define this context include: patient groups (e.g., a positive result on a particular test); conditions of use (e.g., dose and duration of therapy); and a specific therapeutic context (e.g., first- or second-line therapy). Furthermore, in order to define the clinical value of innovation, the estimate of effect of the new drug for the specific clinical context needs to be constrained by the *opportunity cost to the patient* of using the new therapy; the foregone benefits of the best alternative therapy.

4.4.4   Conclusion

Achieving agreement on the clinical value of innovation is only the starting point in the issue of pricing new drugs. The excerpt above from the AUSFTA refers to the need to "appropriately value the objectively demonstrated therapeutic significance of a pharmaceutical". HTA/CEA can provide an objective value of therapeutic significance for a given clinical context (ΔE). It can also provide an objective value of the financial significance of that new drug for a health budget, ΔC, at a particular price (the offer price) of that drug. However, the appropriate value of that new drug in the context of a market transaction, the economic value or shadow price, cannot be derived from the methods developed for HTA/CEA. The concept of shadow price is the subject of the next chapter.

References

AUSPAT (2011) IP Australia. http://pericles.ipaustralia.gov.au/ols/auspat/

Briggs AH, O'Brien BJ (2001) The death of cost-minimization analysis? Health Econ 10(2):179–184

Briggs AH, O'Brien BJ, Blackhouse G (2002) Thinking outside the box: recent advances in the analysis and presentation of uncertainty in cost-effectiveness studies. Annu Rev Public Health 23:377–401

Cohen J, Stolk E, Niezen M (2007) The increasingly complex fourth hurdle for pharmaceuticals. PharmacoEconomics 25(9):727–734

Cook JP, Hunter G, Vernon JA (2009) The future costs, risks and rewards of drug development: the economics of pharmacogenomics. PharmacoEconomics 27(5):355–363. doi:10.2165/00019053-200927050-00001

Davis JC, Furstenthal L, Desai AA, Norris T, Sutaria S, Fleming E, Ma P (2009) The microeconomics of personalized medicine: today's challenge and tomorrow's promise. Nat Rev Drug Discov 8(4):279–286

DeVane C (1994) Pharmacokinetics of the newer antidepressants: clinical relevance. Am J Med 97 (6A):13S–23S

DFAT (2009) Australia-United States Free Trade Agreement, Department of Foreign Affairs and Trade, Australian Government. Available at http://www.dfat.gov.au/fta/ausfta/final-text. Accessed 25 Dec 2013

DiMasi JA (2002) The value of improving the productivity of the drug development process—faster times and better decisions. PharmacoEconomics 20:1–10

FDA (2013) Development and approval process (drugs). http://www.fda.gov/Drugs/DevelopmentApprovalProcess/default.htm. Accessed 25 Dec 2013

Giaccotto C, Santerre RE, Vernon JA (2005) Drug prices and research and development investment behavior in the pharmaceutical industry. J Law Econ 48(1):195–214

O'Brien B (1996) Economic evaluation of pharmaceuticals. Frankenstein's monster or vampire of trials? Med Care Dec 34(12 Suppl):DS99–DS108

PBAC (2013) Guidelines for preparing submissions to the Pharmaceutical Benefits Advisory Committee Version 4.4. http://www.pbac.pbs.gov.au/content/information/printable-files/pbacg-book.pdf. Accessed Dec 2013

Pekarsky BAK (2010) Should financial incentives be used to differentially reward 'me-too' and innovative drugs? PharmacoEconomics 28(1):1–17

Pekarsky BAK (2012) Trust, constraints and the counterfactual: reframing the political economy of new drug price. Dissertation, University of Adelaide. http://digital.library.adelaide.edu.au/dspace/handle/2440/79171. Accessed 25 Dec 2013

Personalized Medicine Coalition (2010) The case for personalized medicine. Available at http://www.personalizedmedicinebulletin.com/wp-content/uploads/sites/205/2011/11/Case_for_PM_3rd_edition1.pdf. Accessed 25 Dec 2013

Pfizer (2011) Pipeline report as of February 28 2011. Available at http://www.pfizer.com/sites/default/files/product-pipeline/pipeline_2011_0228.pdf. Accessed 25 Dec 2012

Pharmaceutical Manufacturing (2013) http://www.pharmamanufacturing.com. Accessed 25 Dec 2013

PhRMA (2011) 2011's new medicines fought wide range of diseases, conditions. Available at www.phrma.org. Accessed at 25 Dec 2011

PhRMA (2013). http://www.phrma.org. Accessed 25 Dec 2013

Temple RJ (2010) Comparative effectiveness research. Available at FDA http://www.fda.gov/downloads/drugs/newsevents/ucm209270.pdf. Accessed 25 Dec 2013

Tirole J (1988) The theory of industrial organization. MIT Press, Cambridge, MA

Trontell A (2010) Comparative effectiveness 101 (with statistical applications). Available at FDA http://www.fda.gov/downloads/Drugs/NewsEvents/UCM209104.pdf. Accessed at Dec 2013

Vernon JA, Golec JH, Lutter R et al (2009) An exploratory study of FDA new drug review times, Prescription Drug User Fee Acts, and R&D spending. Q Rev Econ Finance 49(4):1260–1274

Chapter 5
The Shadow Price, λ

Abstract In countries such as Australia, the UK and Canada, regulators are required to select a decision threshold that is a signal to firms of a price above which the drug is less likely to be purchased. The maximum willingness to pay (maxWTP) for a health effect was the decision threshold preferred by a number of institutions and academics since 1993. In this chapter, the advantages of using a shadow price rather than a maxWTP are demonstrated. These advantages arise because the former necessarily captures information about the forgone benefit of a purchase whereas the latter might or might not. Furthermore, if the price of a substitute good reduces, only the shadow price will reflect the increased competition, not the maxWTP. But which shadow price? There are at least three different shadow prices used in practice, all of which value an action with reference to its minimum possible loss or maximum possible gain. I show that in contexts where there is economic inefficiency and the market fails for a particular input, the derivation of a shadow price for an input from existing information about the economic context (Cost Benefit Analysis, CBA, style) is a more appropriate approach than using the shadow price of a budget constraint. A general method of deriving a CBA-style shadow price for an input without a market price is illustrated.

5.1 The Reimburser's Problem

- How should the objectively determined therapeutic significance of a new drug, its clinical innovation, be valued for the purpose of a market transaction?

The Reimburser recently read a paper by US pharma-economists who stated that the economic value of new drug innovation was indicated by the Payer's maxWTP as revealed by the aICER of the least cost-effective of funded programmes, for example, dialysis (Vernon et al. 2009). Rough calculations suggest to the Reimburser that if all new drugs were paid the aICER of programmes such as dialysis there would be a significant expansion of the current drug budget, and

© Springer International Publishing Switzerland 2015
B.A.K. Pekarsky, *The New Drug Reimbursement Game*,
DOI 10.1007/978-3-319-08903-4_5

health services that are more cost-effective than the new drugs would need to be displaced to finance these additional costs from a fixed health budget.[1]

The Reimburser then reviews a series of papers that refer to the use of the maxWTP as an appropriate value of the health effect, in the absence of evidence of the shadow price of the budget constraint (Johannesson and Weinstein 1993; Stinnett and Mullahy 1998). She also reads a paper by Weinstein (2008) that links the imperative to find a value for a QALY to the recognition by the US population that resources are limited. He argues that the need for a benchmark dollar value of a QALY is present only when a country recognises that it cannot (or will not) afford to buy all citizens effective health care.[2]

Five years ago the Reimburser was involved in the decision to award a significant grant to a group of academics who surveyed over 1,000 people to estimate the maxWTP for a QALY.[3] At the time she was convinced by the argument that because there was no perfectly competitive market for health effects, health tended to be undervalued by the market and therefore it was necessary to survey society to find a value. The Reimburser provides the result of this study (maxWTP per QALY = $75,000) to her Health Economic Adviser as a guide to the economic value of the health effects of a new drug. The Reimburser is confused when the Health Economic Adviser states that this information is not what he needs. The Health Economic Adviser uses this example to illustrate the issue:

> A Consumer asks her Agent to purchase a particular new bicycle on her behalf. Which of the two following pieces of information should she give her Agent? The maximum price she is willing to pay for the bicycle ($5,000) or the lowest price that bicycle is available for, according to the results of an online search ($1,250)? The latter is the shadow price of the bike, the former is the maxWTP.

The Reimburser is inclined to say the shadow price is the price the Consumer should give her Agent. In fact, if the market for this type of bike were perfectly competitive, then it would not matter which of these two prices the Consumer gave her Agent. In this case the price at every shop would be $1,250 and hence the price the Agent pays for a new bike would be $1,250, regardless of the information the Agent is provided with and regardless of the Consumer's maxWTP. However, if the local market were a monopoly and the online price were from a competitive market, then it *would* matter which price she gave her Agent; the monopolist could be pricing at average rather than marginal cost and hence the purchase price could be

---

[1] See Pekarsky (2012, Appendix 7) for a discussion the issue of choice of the aICER and full value price in more detail.

[2] See page 345 in Weinstein (2008).

[3] The inspiration for the study was one very similar to that described in Donaldson et al. (2011).

higher than the online price from a competitive market. The potential loss resulting from providing the wrong piece of information to her Agent would be maximised under the following scenario.

> The local monopolist bike shop owner does not provide price tags for her new bikes. Instead she asks the Agent, what is the maximum you are willing to pay for a bike? Then, after receiving this information she writes a price tag for that bike and offers it to the Agent. In this case the Agent would pay $5,000 for the bike if the only information that were provided to the Agent was the maxWTP. The loss of surplus to the Consumer would be $3,750 (=$5,000 − $1,250). If the Agent were provided with the information about the shadow price, and the local monopolist bike shop owner knew the Agent could take her business elsewhere (not such a monopoly after all), she would have reduced this price.

This example makes the intended point, but it just does not seem "technical enough" to the Reimburser. There is no "online price" from a competitive market for a new drug against which she can benchmark the new drug price. The Reimburser asks her Health Economic Adviser:

- Why is it that the maxWTP is not an economic value?
- Which shadow price should she use?

5.2   Why Is the Shadow Price Preferable to the maxWTP?

The key difference between the shadow price and the maxWTP is that the former acts as a conventional price by capturing information about the economic context (albeit imperfectly) whereas the maxWTP captures only one aspect of the economic context, the consumer's preferences. If there is increased competition in the market for a good and its substitutes, the maxWTP for the item does not change, whereas the shadow price will reduce.

A hypothetical application of shadow prices to a real world problem (the non-excludability and non-rivalry of the outputs of dung beetles) illustrates this issue. The method is an adaption of those described by Mishan and Quah (2007) and McKean (1972).

5.2.1   Dung Beetles, Flies and Outdoor Dining in Canberra

When the number of flies in Australia was reduced by the introduction of dung beetles by the Australian Commonwealth Scientific and Industrial Research

Organisation (CSIRO) in the 1980s, outdoor dining in places such as Canberra became possible, apparently for the first time. There is no dung beetle market in Australia, despite their tangible and significant value to the Australian economy (Commonwealth Scientific and Industrial Research Organisation 2006). The output of a programme to introduce dung beetles is both non-rival in consumption and non-excludable; such a programme is a public good. So how can we derive a price for the main input into this programme; the dung beetle? (While the role of dung beetles in reducing flies in Canberra is true, the following story about the bidding process and competition is completely fictional.)

Assume for the sake of simplicity that the only output of the dung beetle programme is fly-free outdoor dining in Canberra (FFODC). Assume that there are three inputs in this programme, two of which are priced at their marginal cost of production (transport and labour) and one of which does not have a price (the dung beetle). Now assume that there is an alternative method for achieving FFODC and there is a functioning market for this good (outdoor fly screens). The evidence of the value in exchange of FFODC is revealed in the functioning market of outdoor fly screens.

This story is set out in Tables 5.1 to 5.5. The Canberra Council, which will finance this dung beetle programme, wants to know about its costs. CSIRO is the only group in Australia to have a licence to import dung beetles and there is no other way for the Canberra Council to obtain them.

Part 1 From the first column of Table 5.1, we see that the labour and transport costs for the dung beetle programme are $100 thousand and $10 thousand respectively. CSIRO has not told the Canberra Council how much it costs for the 1,000 dung beetles. CSIRO has also financed a rigorous study that estimated the maxWTP by the Canberra population for the state of FFODC and found this was an amount of $20 million. The Council asks the CSIRO the cost of the dung beetles. They reply that it is $19,890 per beetle or $20 million for the overall cost of the program. This is exactly the maxWTP for FFODC. The owners of the Outdoor Fly Screen Company make an urgent submission to Canberra Council. They say they can achieve the same result (FFODC) with a different programme for $1.15 million (Table 5.2). Clearly, even though the cost of the dung beetle programme is the same as the benefits, there is a more cost-effective option. The Canberra Council decides to use outdoor fly screens.

Part 2 CSIRO comes back to the Council and says they have revised their costs. They can now provide dung beetles for $1,040 each (Part 2, Table 5.1). The costs of the dung beetle programme are now the same as the outdoor fly screen programme: $1.15 million.

This simple example illustrates the following point. If there is only one situation in which dung beetles are an input, and there is a failure of a dung beetle market to function, then, provided that there are multiple inputs and methods of production that can be used to achieve the same output (FFODC), a shadow price for dung beetles that takes into account this competition can be calculated. The dung beetle is valued at $19,890 but its shadow price is $1,040.

Table 5.1 Cost of dung beetle programme

	Part 1	Part 2	Scenario
	Max WTP output	Shadow price input	Max WTP output (higher costs of production for dung beetle programme)
Labour	$100,000	$100,000	$2,000,000
Transport	$10,000	$10,000	$30,000
Subtotal	$110,000	$110,000	$2,030,000
Dung beetles—no market price			
1,000 beetles	$19,890,000	$1,040,000	$17,970,000
Per beetle	$19,890	$1,040	$17,970
Programme total cost	$20,000,000	$1,150,000	$20,000,000

The price charged for dung beetles varies across parts and scenario.

Table 5.2 Cost of outdoor fly screen programme

	Part 1	Part 2	Scenario
	Max WTP output	Shadow price input	Max WTP output (higher costs of manufacture for dung beetle programme)
Labour	$100,000	$100,000	$100,000
Transport	$50,000	$50,000	$50,000
Fly screens	$1,000,000	$1,000,000	$1,000,000
Programme total cost	$1,150,000	$1,150,000	$1,150,000

The results do not vary across parts and scenario; they are not dependent upon dung beetle price.

Table 5.3 Maximum willingness to pay for fly free outdoor dining

	Part 1	Part 2	Scenario
	Max WTP output	Shadow price input	Max WTP output (higher costs of manufacture for dung beetle program)
Max WTP	$20,000,000	$20,000,000	$20,000,000

The results do not vary across parts and scenario; they are not dependent upon dung beetle price.

So why is it that there is an advantage to the Canberra Council in using the shadow price? The first advantage is that if outdoor fly screens are a more cost-effective way to achieve the intended output of outdoor dining, Canberra's Council will recognise that they can achieve the same result at a much lower cost. The maxWTP considers only the preferences for outdoor dining and not alternative method of achieving this; it values the output rather than the specific input.

The second advantage of this approach is that it maximises consumer welfare. CSIRO knows the maxWTP for the benefits of the programme; it conducted the study to estimate it. If the CSIRO knew that the competition (fly screens) was not

Table 5.4 The social welfare impact of implementing the dung beetle programme*

	Part 1	Part 2	Scenario
	Max WTP output	Shadow price input	Max WTP output (higher costs of manufacture for dung beetle program)
Cost of dung beetle programme	$20,000,000	$1,150,000	$20,000,000
Surplus (MaxWTP less cost)	$19,890,000	$19,890,000	$17,970,000
Dung beetle patent holder	$19,890,000	$1,040,000	$17,970,000
Consumer surplus	$0	$18,850,000	$0
Deadweight loss	$0	$0	$880,000

The results vary across parts and scenario due to the different ways the drug beetle price is selected

Table 5.5 The social welfare impact of implementing the outdoor fly screen programme

	Part 1	Part 2	Scenario
	Max WTP output	Shadow price input	Max WTP output (higher costs of manufacture for dung beetle program)
Cost of outdoor fly screen programme	$1,150,000	$1,150,000	$1,150,000
Surplus (MaxWTP less cost)	$18,850,000	$18,850,000	$18,850,000
Consumer surplus	$18,850,000	$18,850,000	$18,850,000

Result does not vary across parts and scenarios as it does not depend on dung beetle price

recognised, then it would be possible for the CSIRO to appropriate the entire surplus associated with the reduction in flies in Canberra by pricing its input such that the total cost of the programme is the same as the maxWTP. At the shadow price the surplus is appropriated by the consumers. The point is that not only does the shadow price capture information about the economic context—the competition in the outdoor dining market—it also has the potential to reduce the risks associated with other distortions that could arise as a consequence of, for example, market power due to patents.

The third problem this method overcomes is the deadweight loss[4] that can arise when the maxWTP for the output is used to derive the price of an input with market power and the competition of the alternative input is neglected. The Scenario columns from Tables 5.1 to 5.5 illustrate an example where the financial costs of labour and transport for the dung beetle programme are higher than the total costs of the outdoor fly screen programme. Even if the benefits outweigh the costs of the dung beetle programme, for example it could be priced at $15 million, there could

---

[4] There is a reduction in social surplus, not just a redistribution of surplus; even if one subgroup is better off, the entire group is worse off.

still be a deadweight loss of \$880,000 compared with the best alternative strategy, the outdoor fly screen programme.

The observable difference between a value for the dung beetle calculated using the maxWTP for FFODC rather than a shadow price for that effect is as follows. The maxWTP for output-derived value of the dung beetle as an input remains constant, regardless of how much competition there is to produce that output. The method can tell us what the dung beetle is worth from a lay perspective, but not its economic value. In contrast, the shadow price for that dung beetle (derived from the shadow price for the input, which is in turn derived from a functioning market) is defined by the economic environment, and will change as competition in the input markets changes. The shadow price tells us what the Canberra Council should pay for a dung beetle given the competition in the market. It also maximises consumer surplus and prevents deadweight losses in social welfare.

The shadow price for the dung beetle is *endogenous* to the economic context (the market for reduction in number of flies in outdoor dining areas). The value of the dung beetle derived using the maxWTP is *exogenous* to the economic context; it reveals the consumer's preferences which are not subjected to the constraints of alternative methods of producing the outcome of reduced flies. The shadow price of that input, unlike its maxWTP,[5] internalises the economic conditions, albeit with varying degrees of consistency between the specified economic context and the real world economic context.

We can conclude that shadow prices are preferable to maxWTP to value an input, particularly when there is competition in the market for inputs and the input being valued has market power. However, there is more than one type of shadow price. So which shadow price should be used in the context of the economic value of pharmaceutical innovation?

5.3   Shadow Prices

The key concept of a shadow price is that the value of a resource allocation action is defined objectively by reference to its minimum possible loss or maximum possible gain. In the case of the dung beetles, the shadow price is defined with reference to the best alternative fly reduction strategy and will increase and decrease as the costs of the alternative change. However, there is more than one type of shadow price referred to in the economic literature. In the most recent edition of the 1971 classic text on cost benefit analysis (Mishan 1971), Mishan and Quah (2007) identified two usages of the term shadow price in the context of general economics and these are discussed below. Other authors have discussed the issue of finite divisibility of

---

[5] The maxWTP is not immune to changes in context for example, when it rains, the price of umbrellas night increase.

programmes and the implications for shadow price and decision rules and hence a third usage of the term "shadow price" by Kim and Cho (1988) is also discussed.

5.3.1   Three Shadow Prices

The first usage of "shadow price" identified by Mishan and Quah (2007) is in the context of optimisation techniques and it differs slightly in its definition in economics compared to operations research. In operations research, the shadow price is the *minimum* loss in effect that occurs when one unit of a continuous resource (or constraint) is *withdrawn* (Takayama 1994). In economics, it is the *maximum* additional units of maximand or effect gained as a consequence of *relaxing* a constraint by one unit at the margin. The value of the Lagrange multiplier, λ, at optimisation is an example of this type of shadow price (Mas-Colell et al. 1995).[6][7] The shadow price, λ, in this context is also referred to as the shadow price of the budget constraint; this is the sense in which the term is used by a number of health economists.[8]

The second usage identified by Mishan and Quah is in the context of a CBA. The definition proposed by Mishan and Quah is the appropriate price for an input or output in the context of CBA when the market price does not reflect the true social cost or benefit. One example is when the market price is systematically failing to include some aspect of the cost or benefit of the production or consumption of a good or service, e.g., the externality of pollution. Shadow prices are also used when there is no apparent market for a particular input or output. An example of the use of shadow price in this sense is the valuation of volunteer or carer time in a HTA/CEA.[9][10]

---

[6] The shadow price can also be defined in an examination of the first order conditions required for Pareto optimality. It can be defined as the multiplier derived from the Kuhn-Tucker theory at optimality—it is the additional utility to a consumer as a consequence of relaxing an endowment constraint. See for example (Mas-Colell et al. 1995) page 563.

[7] If there were decreasing marginal returns to additional inputs or resources we would expect that a shadow price that was derived using the operations research definition would be greater than that derived using the economic definition.

[8] See for example Stinnett and Mullahy(1998) and Sendi et al. (2002).

[9] See for example Drummond et al. (2005) pages 58–59.

[10] Sculpher et al. (2005) appear to characterise shadow pricing as exclusively defined within and applying to a first best world and hence the limits on using shadow pricing can be inferred as equivalent to the limits of assuming a first best world. The authors argue that neoclassical welfare economic theory is an "application to a presumed nirvana of a first-best neoclassical world" despite it clearly not being a world in which market prices do not represent social opportunity cost nor can these goods and services be shadow priced in this world. The authors use this argument as a justification for their preference for a social decision making rather than neoclassical welfare economic theory as a foundation to economic evaluation of health care technologies. The capacity to develop a shadow price for a good within welfare economic theory and attempt to take

In addition to the two uses identified by Mishan and Quah, shadow price has particular meaning in operations research and decision analysis in cases where the inputs are integer or discrete rather than continuous (Kim and Cho 1988). Mukherjee and Chatterjee state that these authors, by introducing the concept of an average shadow price, gave a "valid economic interpretation" to the shadow price for integer programming (Mukherjee and Chatterjee 2006 p. 13).

The concept of an average shadow price as a critical price above which there is no incentive to purchase a discrete input is of relevance to health economics; in a universal health care system, decisions regarding new technologies tend to be in relation to financing the technology for no patients or for all patients in a particular target group. Kim and Cho's definition of a shadow price is in the same units as the CBA shadow price (cost per unit output rather than units of output as in the optimisation context); however, its application to decision-making is different. In this case it is applied as a threshold or critical price in the context of a decision by a firm to acquire a discrete input, rather than as a shadow price of a given input or output to be used in a CBA and an associated metric such as a Cost Benefit ratio. In this way it has the potential to become a signal to the owner of that input, instead of the more passive[11] approach to costing inherent in a CBA.

It would appear that when CBA methods use the concept of a shadow price of an input, it is being used to refer to an average shadow price rather than a marginal shadow price; projects valued by CBA (and therefore their inputs) are often discrete rather than continuous. But the use of the term "average shadow price" rather than a marginal shadow price can lead to some discomfort for economists. Why? And does it matter?

5.3.1.1   Why Should We Be as Comfortable to Use an Average as a Marginal Shadow Price?

In the context of new drug reimbursement policies, which are discrete, the concept of an average shadow price is more appropriate than a marginal shadow price.[12] However, the concept of a marginal shadow price dominates the literature, and the term shadow price therefore tends to be interpreted by economists as a marginal

---

into account market failure is not explored by these authors. It is likely (but not certain) that the authors' argument is an extension (or characterisation or application) of the debate between Mishan and Williams, one side of which is expounded in Mishan (1982). It would be useful to reduce the uncertainty surrounding the rationale of their decision to use this as a justification.

[11] In the health economic literature, the cost in a CBA is generally accepted as a given or an attempt is made to adjust it to reflect a social opportunity cost, but it is not seen as a signal to the producer of the value in exchange of that input. For example, see Chap. 7 in Drummond et al. (2005).

[12] Weinstein and Stason (1976) seems to be the earliest reference used in the health economic literature to refer to the discrete properties of health programs and the implications for optimal allocation of health resources. Birch and Gafni (1992) is probably a better known reference and discussed the implications for shadow prices and budget constraints.

concept. Is it because marginal is the "correct" concept and average is "incorrect"? Is it the case of an expanding margin? Or is it because the marginal shadow price is derived from a model that has good properties for theory but not for applied economics? Is it legitimate to rely on an average rather than marginal shadow price in the context of the reimbursement decision?

The key role of a shadow price is to put a price on any constraint by referencing this to the potential gain or loss from changing this constraint. The simplest models from which a shadow price can be derived as part of the optimisation problem are those that are continuously differentiable and hence all inputs and outputs are continuous (infinitely divisible). In this way, first order conditions and a unique solution (if there is one) to the optimisation problem can be identified. The theoretical advantages of a continuously differentiable function are well appreciated.[13] However, one only needs to look at the extraordinarily strict conditions that need to be met in order to have well behaved utility functions to be reminded of the key trade-off in a theoretical model: the better behaved the model, the less relevant to the real world.[14]

The linear programming problem with continuously differentiable functions is the operations research equivalent of a well behaved utility function with neat solutions. One real world adaptation of such a problem is the introduction of discrete inputs. When the inputs are discrete, the function(s) is no longer continuously differentiable. The relevance of integer or mixed programming in health economics was identified in Birch and Gafni (1992). As Kim and Cho (1988) demonstrate, the process of finding the optimal allocation of resources becomes much more complex when discrete inputs are introduced (but the leap in complexity is probably less of an issue given the improvements in computational tools since 1988). With developments in software and processing power, the complexity of solving problems is reduced, but the information requirements for using integer programming to solve resource allocation problems for entire budgets remain significant. However, the constraint placed on the set of optimal solutions by removing the condition of a continuous function is a necessary attribute of a model that captures this significant real world characteristic.

The dung beetle example adds one additional layer of complexity to this mixed programming problem: prices are not available for one input and there is the potential for market power. If the problem were to optimally allocate all of Canberra Local Government's resources across possible opportunities to improve

---

[13] For example, many neoclassical macroeconomic problems start with the Inada conditions about a production function of a firm. These conditions are necessary to ensure that in a neoclassical growth model, the growth path is stable. There are six conditions, one of which is that the function is continuously differential, which in turn implies that the inputs are continuous and not "lumpy" (Hahn 2008). Cobb Douglas production functions also meet the condition of being continuously differentiable (Brown 2008).

[14] Most advanced microeconomic text books will detail these conditions. See for example Jehle and Reny (2001) Sect. 1.3, the Consumers Problem in particular, Theorem 1.4 on the sufficiency of the consumer's first order conditions.

the welfare of its citizens, then the task would be prohibitively complex, regardless of whether linear or integer programming were used. However, by partialising the problem to the objective of reducing the number of flies in Canberra, the constraint that provides the shadow price is the best alternative use of resources to achieve this outcome. However, the shadow price in this case is an average shadow price because even though we can choose to use outdoor fly screens at one or 100 outdoor restaurants, the dung beetle programme has discrete properties; it is either implemented or not, and if implemented requires a minimum number of beetles to become a self-sustaining programme. The decision is not how big the programme should be; it is how much the Council should pay for it.

In conclusion, whether an average or marginal shadow price is the most appropriate solution concept for a problem is a characteristic of the structure of the problem. The average shadow price is the best way to price a constraint in problems such as those described by Kim and Cho and the Canberra fly reduction problem. It is possible that the marginal shadow price is the dominant concept in the economic literature as a consequence of theoreticians' and teachers' rational preference for a continuously differential function in order to demonstrate a key economic principle; the necessity of defining an opportunity cost in order to achieve optimisation. When discrete inputs are introduced, the overall optimisation problem becomes more complex, but the fact that the shadow price is average not marginal is the inevitable result of the structure of the problem, not a methodological choice.

5.3.2 How Does the Value of a Given Shadow Price Respond to Economic Contexts?

One difference between types of shadow prices is their relevance in a context of economic inefficiency, market power and the resultant price distortions. If the budget is not economically efficient then the shadow price of the budget constraint is not necessarily representative of the (full or potential) economic value of an expanded or contracted budget.

Consider the example of a budget for public transport. Assume that the least cost-effective currently funded mode of transport (e.g., diesel buses costing $100 per 100 km) is less cost-effective than the most cost-effective unfunded mode of transport (e.g., electric buses at $50 per 100 km). There is an opportunity to improve the output for a given budget by reallocating funds from the funded to the unfunded programme. In this case, if the shadow price of contracting the existing budget were calculated before achieving economic efficiency, it would yield a lower economic value of the budget (1 km lost per reduction in budget of $1) than if calculated after achieving economic efficiency (2 km lost per reduction in budget of $1). This situation is analogous to the bias that would occur if the clinical value of innovation were defined by using health gains of the least effective available alternative therapy instead of the foregone benefits of the most effective alternative existing therapy.

Significantly, in CBA, the use of the concept of "shadow price" as a price for an input is intended to be a solution to the problem of valuing inputs and outputs in a way that reflects economic constraints in a situation where there is market failure that leads to inefficiency. In many cases this market failure is the motivation for using CBA.[15] The use of the shadow price in this context requires that the analyst understands the many sources of market failure in the current situation. In contrast, the shadow price as the marginal unit lost or gained when the budget is tightened or relaxed in a linear programing problem is only relevant when the budget is economically efficient and the markets are perfectly competitive.[16] It does not require that the analyst explore sources of market failure because it assumes there are none.

5.3.2.1   Derive the Input Price from the maxWTP for the Output or the Shadow Price for the Output

There are two ways a price for an input without a market price can be derived and applied. First, we could derive the input's value from a maxWTP for the output. Second, we could derive the input's price from the shadow price of the output. These options correspond to Parts 1 and 2 from the dung beetle programme example. They also correspond to a choice by the Reimburser: should the price for the new drug be derived from the maxWTP for the output or the shadow price for that output? Hence we ask: which of these two methods achieves an "appropriate" economic value of the clinical innovation of a new drug? Clearly, if a new drug had a competitive market price then we would not need to have an annex to the AUSFTA to set the parameters for such a price. Also, market power is a characteristic of the market for new drugs. Furthermore, budgets are fixed or constrained and there is significant competition in the health input market. Hence the derivation of an appropriate price for the new drug in the context of the market transaction called "reimbursement" is most appropriately generated from a shadow price for the most cost-effective strategy of achieving health gains for any group in a population with any health inputs. And finally, as demonstrated in the dung beetle

---

[15] So why is there a preference for maximum willingness to pay as a way of valuing the benefits in a CBA? [For example see Sugden and Williams (1978) and Drummond et al. (2005).] The dung beetle example presented in this Chapter shows how if the maxWTP is used to value the output of the dung beetle and then to price the dung beetle, particularly when there is market power, and there is competition in means of producing the output. Essentially we can separate out the valuation of the surplus from the question of the allocation of that surplus across producer and consumer by introducing the competing use of resources, the outdoor fly screens. This issue seems to me to be one of the sources of tension between Williams and Mishan as described by Mishan (1982).

[16] This situation is explored in detail in Chap. 5.

example, the appropriately derived shadow price of the output can be used as a signal to firms supplying inputs, hence the shadow price for that input can be derived by the supplier and the average shadow price of the output becomes a decision threshold for the purchaser.

Do health economists use shadow price in this way to value a new drug? No, not at this stage, but they do use shadow price in a number of ways.

5.4   Shadow Price and Health Economics

The majority of the health economic literature on the topic of the shadow price and the associated areas of CBA and decision thresholds appears to have its origins in Sugden and Williams (1978) and the seminal paper from Weinstein and Zeckhauser (1973). The reliance on this stream of literature is unsurprising given the significant roles that Williams and Weinstein played in the development of health economics in the UK and the US respectively. However, these authors have very little overlap with the stream of literature that applies shadow price in the CBA context using methods described by Mishan and Quah (2007) and McKean (1972).[17] Possibly as a consequence of these origins, and its close association in operations research methods,[18] the health economic literature generally uses the term "shadow price" to refer to the shadow price of the budget constraint (Stinnett and Mullahy 1998)or to the valuation of an input such as voluntary carer time, for which there is a supply but no market price (Coupé et al. 2007). There is some discussion about the shadow price of capital and its relationship to the discount rate (Drummond et al. (2005)). There is also a significant amount of literature on the question of the valuation of health gains for the purpose of a CBA. This valuation tends to be based on consumer or social preferences for health, and does not take into consideration competing means of producing these outcomes.[19]

Most authors recognise the practical limitations of using the shadow price of the budget constraint as a decision threshold for new drugs or any other programme. The challenge has become to find a reasonable substitute. For example, in a paper that argues for the routine use of a second best rule to opportunity cost in assessing decisions about programmes, Sendi et al. (2002) identify the shadow price as having a relationship with the decision threshold and as an indicator of value in the absence of a market: *The threshold value λ reflects the shadow price per unit effectiveness (e.g. dollars per life-years saved) in the absence of a market.*

---

[17] A paper by O'Brien and Gafni(1996) does apply Mishan's methods of contingent valuation to the health outputs of a health program, however it does not address the issue of valuing inputs with market power. It does address the issue of analysing the relationship between price and demand in a private market for health services as a way of valuing health.

[18] Pharmaco-economic models are often developed by operations researchers (applied mathematicians) in conjunction with economists.

[19] For example, see Chap. 7 in Drummond et al. (2005).

The authors then go on to discuss a number of factors that could constrain the use of this shadow price as the threshold in programme adoption, including: being unable to quantify λ if the budget constraint is not defined from a societal perspective; the finite divisibility of health resources and programmes; and the stochastic nature of the evidence of the marginal programme and hence the shadow price. The authors advocate the use of the average ICER[20] of displaced services as a second best alternative to the shadow price of the budget constraint, with a particular emphasis on the point that the average ICER of the service displaced is a function of program size.

Some authors have developed shadow prices in the sense of valuing a good or service for which there is no market. Van den Berg used multiple methods to value informal care, including contingent valuation and willingness to pay and accept. He also explored the psychological effects of monetisation of informal care (Van den Berg 2005).

The idea that charges for services do not necessarily represent their "cost" has a long history.[21] This debate is typically made with reference to internal prices set by organisations and there is an extensive discussion in Drummond et al. (2005) in relation to the question of costing non-market inputs in the absence of a market price. However, there appears to be a reluctance to consider the implications of using a price that is set in a market where there is significant market power, for example specialists and medical technologies. Drummond et al. (2005) indicate that the issue of the difference between market prices of inputs and their opportunity cost is well known amongst health economists. In a discussion of whether or not the price of an input should be accepted even though in cases such as a new drugs it is unlikely to be indicative of its social opportunity cost, the authors conclude that "market imperfections" are only recognised by health economists if they are undertaking an evaluation. They argue that adjustments for these imperfections should only occur if otherwise "substantial bias" enters the study and the adjustment can be made using a "clear and objective" method (Drummond et al. 2005 p. 58). The authors do not go on to propose a rigorous method whereby this adjusted price could be derived.

It can be concluded that most health economists are familiar with the idea of a shadow price, however, it seems that they are less likely to be familiar with its

---

[20] The concept of an average ICER for displaced services takes into account the fact that if the amount of services that are displaced changes, then the aICER could change if there are increasing or decreasing marginal costs.

[21] McNeil et al. (1975) is an example of this history. While there were some earlier discussions about this issue in the literature, this discussion of the issue is particularly eloquent. The paper makes no reference to the question of market power of the patent holders of the new technology; an omission typical of most cost-effectiveness analyses. The paper does refers to the idea that even if the new technology is cost-effective that this is not sufficient information to justify its adoption because budgetary implications also need to be considered. That particular edition of the New England Journal of Medicine was a microcosm of the critical issues in health economics and Bayesian statistics at that time.

application in CBA as described by Mishan and Quah (2007) and McKean (1972) than they are with the applications by Sugden and Williams (1978) and Weinstein and Zeckhauser(1973). This asymmetry in understanding limits the historic application of shadow pricing in health economics, but it also highlights an opportunity for further development.

5.5 Discussion and Conclusion

Health economists always recognised the significance of a shadow price of a budget constraint as the ideal decision threshold against which the results of economic evaluations (the ICER) can be benchmarked and the decision to allocate resources to a program informed. The impracticalities of using the shadow price of the budget constraint are also widely recognised. Health economists have been quick to point out situations where the market price fails to accommodate the full value of health benefits and there is a long tradition of valuing health outcomes using the maxWTP. However, as shown in the example of the dung beetle program, the use of maxWTP for an output to derive a value for an input, when that input has market power, can have significant implications for consumer surplus and for a potential deadweight loss.

Health economic textbooks indicate a need for methods to value inputs appropriately but do not propose "*clear and objective ways of making the adjustment*" to a market price where this market price is likely to reflect market power. The welfare economic literature does provide a suitable starting point. Examples of general methods to derive the shadow price of an input are set out in Mishan and Quah (2007) and McKean (1972).[22] The key issue is to recognise that the constraint to the adoption of this input (for example the dung beetle) is the best alternative input (the outdoor fly screens) and that the shadow price represents this constraint.

In summary, the health economic focus on the shadow price of the budget constraint as *the* shadow price relevant to health care decisions can lead to the following Catch 22: we can't find this shadow price until economic efficiency is achieved and we can't improve economic efficiency until this price is found. Chapter 6 introduces a method, PEA, whereby such a shadow price can be developed in the context of a reimbursement process. The imperative of PEA is to find a shadow price for health effects that will improve economic efficiency rather than one that is conditional on economic efficiency. This is consistent with the role of a shadow price in the welfare economic literature in the tradition of Mishan and McKean.

---

[22] In pages 135–139, McKean sets out three method to derive the shadow price of an input by using information available from other decisions and other "price relationships observed in other markets for similar items" (McKean 1972).

References

Brown M (2008) Cobb-Douglas functions. In: Durlauf SN, Blume LE (eds) The New Palgrave dictionary of economics. Palgrave Macmillan, Basingstoke

Birch S, Gafni A (1992) Cost-effectiveness/utility analyses: do current decision rules lead us to where we want to be? J Health Econ 11(3):279–296

Commonwealth Scientific and Industrial Research Organisation (2006) Dung beetles. http://www.csiro.au/resources/DungBeetles.html. Accessed 25 Dec 2013

Coupé V, Veenhof C, Van Tulder M, Dekker J, Bijlsma J, Van den Ende C (2007) The cost-effectiveness of behavioural graded activity in patients with osteoarthritis of hip and/or knee. Ann Rheum Dis 66(2):215–221

Donaldson C, Baker R, Mason H, Jones-Lee M, Lancsar E, Wildman J, Bateman I, Loomes G, Robinson A, Sugden R, Prades J, Ryan M, Shackley P, Smith R (2011) The social value of a QALY: raising the bar or barring the raise? BMC Health Serv Res 11(1):8

Drummond MF, Sculpher MJ, Torrance GW, O'Brien BJ, Stoddart GL (2005) Methods for the economic evaluation of health care programmes, 3rd edn. Oxford University Press, Oxford

Hahn FH (2008) Neoclassical growth theory. In: Durlauf SN, Blume LE (eds) The New Palgrave dictionary of economics. Palgrave Macmillan, Basingstoke

Jehle G, Reny P (2001) Advanced microeconomic theory, 2nd edn. Addison Wesley, Boston

Johannesson M, Weinstein MC (1993) On the decision rules of cost-effectiveness analysis. J Health Econ 12(4):459–467

Kim S, Cho SC (1988) A shadow price in integer programming for management decision. Eur J Oper Res 37(3):328–335

Mas-Colell A, Whinston M, Green J (1995) Microeconomic theory. Oxford University Press, New York

McKean RN (1972) The use of shadow prices. In: Layard R (ed) Cost benefit analysis. Penguin, Harmondsworth, pp 119–139

McNeil BJ, Varady PD, Burrows BA, Adelstein SJ (1975) Cost-effectiveness calculations in the diagnosis and treatment of hypertensive renovascular disease. N Engl J Med 293(5):216–221

Mishan E (1971) Cost-benefit analysis: an informal introduction. Allen & Unwin, London

Mishan E (1982) The new controversy about the rationale of economic evaluation. J Econ Issues XVI(1):29–47

Mishan E, Quah E (2007) Cost-benefit analysis, 5th edn. Routledge, Abingdon

Mukherjee S, Chatterjee A (2006) Unified concept of bottleneck. Working Paper series of IIMA. Indian Institute of Management, Bangalore

O'Brien B, Gafni A (1996) When do the "dollars" make sense? Med Decis Mak 16:288–299

Pekarsky BAK (2012) Trust, constraints and the counterfactual: reframing the political economy of new drug price. Dissertation, University of Adelaide. http://digital.library.adelaide.edu.au/dspace/handle/2440/79171. Accessed 25 Dec 2013

Sculpher M, Claxton K, Akehurst R (2005) It's just evaluation for decision-making: recent developments in, and challenges for, cost-effectiveness research. In: Smith P, Ginnelly L, Sculpher M (eds) Health policy and economics: opportunities and challenges. Open University Press, Maidenhead, pp 8–41

Sendi P, Gafni A, Birch S (2002) Opportunity costs and uncertainty in the economic evaluation of health care interventions. Health Econ 11(1):23–31

Stinnett AA, Mullahy J (1998) Net health benefits: a new framework for the analysis of uncertainty in cost-effectiveness analysis. Med Decis Mak 18(2):S68–S80

Sugden R, Williams A (1978) The principles of practical cost-benefit analysis. Oxford University Press, Oxford

Takayama A (1994) Analytical methods in economics. Harvester Wheatsheaf, Hemel

Van den Berg R (2005) Informal care: an economic approach. Erasmus University, Rotterdamn

Vernon JA, Goldberg R, Golec JH (2009) Economic evaluation and cost-effectiveness thresholds: signals to firms and implications for R & D investment and innovation. PharmacoEconomics 27(10):797–806

Weinstein MC (2008) How much are Americans willing to pay for a quality-adjusted life year? Med Care 46(4):343–345

Weinstein MC, Stason WB (1976) Hypertension: a policy perspective. Harvard University Press, Cambridge, MA

Weinstein MC, Zeckhauser RJ (1973) Critical ratios and efficient allocation. J Public Econ 2 (2):147–157

Part II
The New Drug Decision Threshold

Chapter 6
The Health Shadow Price, β_c

Abstract This chapter introduces five concepts central to this book. The *opportunity cost of a strategy in an institutional setting* is identified when the decision maker values all states of the world that could emerge under different allocations of resources, not just the alternative options available to her or him. *Price-effectiveness analysis* is a method of assessing the decision to reimburse a new drug by testing the relationship between the incremental price-effectiveness ratio (IPER) of the new drug and the population's health. The *strategy of reimbursement* comprises the actions of adoption and financing. The *health shadow price, β_c* is the IPER of the health effects gained by the target patients as a consequence of the strategy of reimbursing (adopting and financing) the new drug with clinical innovation and additional financial cost such that the funder is indifferent between the strategy of reimbursement and the best alternative strategy available to the funder using the same financial resources. The *economic value of clinical innovation* (EVCI) is the gross clinical benefit of the new drug, constrained twice: by the clinical opportunity cost (the best alternative therapy to the new drug) and the economic opportunity cost (the best alternative use of resources). The health shadow price β_c and EVCI are derived for the case of an economically efficient fixed budget with no failure in the market for health inputs.

6.1 The Reimburser's Problem

The Reimburser understands that the choice of the decision threshold for a new drug is a complex one, both technically and politically. She also understands it is related to the idea of the appropriate valuation in a market context of the objectively determined therapeutic significance of a new drug. After discussions with her Health Economic Adviser about clinical innovation and the shadow price she decides that what she needs is an average shadow price for the health effects from the new drug, which is expressed as a decision threshold and is calculated with reference to the best alternative use of the incremental financial cost of the new drug, ΔC (Chap. 5). A firm can then use this information as a signal of the

© Springer International Publishing Switzerland 2015
B.A.K. Pekarsky, *The New Drug Reimbursement Game*,
DOI 10.1007/978-3-319-08903-4_6

maximum acceptable IPER of the new drug. But how should she arrive at such a measure? The Reimburser asks her Health Economic Adviser:

- Is there a shadow price for the health effects of a new drug that:
  - Is based on the opportunity cost of the best alternative way to produce health effects;
  - Can be used as a decision threshold IPER for a new drug; and
  - Is sensitive to the economic context?

6.2   The Path to the Health Shadow Price

The Health Economic Adviser provides the Reimburser with the path that he used to develop the idea of the objective value of the health effects of a new drug, the health shadow price. This path is illustrated in Fig 6.1. The Reimburser works her way along this path, starting with the question of the appropriate value of "the objectively demonstrated therapeutic significance of a pharmaceutical". The Reimburser recognises that this is about the value of the clinical innovation in the context of an economic transaction, where the patent holder (the firm) has market power. However, as a large monopsonist purchaser, she also has some market power. In this situation she can choose to value the new drug using either an economic concept (opportunity cost) or a lay concept (value for money) that does not recognise the economic context. The former is preferable to the latter in this context.

The opportunity cost of reimbursing a new drug is not what is physically displaced to finance the new drug; that is an operational issue. The opportunity cost is the best alternative strategy to reimbursement. Furthermore, as a member of an institution, the Reimburser does not need to focus only on alternative strategies physically available to her. According to Buchanan (2008), in an institutional setting, the use of the term "opportunity cost to the decision" does not necessarily imply that the decision maker is physically choosing between these two strategies and their corresponding end-state alternatives. Instead, it means that the decision maker is valuing all states of the world that could emerge under different allocations of resources, in this case, the resources with a financial value of ΔC. This definition overcomes, at some level at least, the possible failure of the institution to include these alternatives in the physical choice set; in particular, unpatented services such as workforce strategies, respite care and training of health workers.[1]

---

[1] From the New Palgrave Dictionary of Economics, Buchanan's definition of opportunity cost in the institutional setting emphasises the significance of considering strategies that might lead to outcomes that are not possible from strategies that are considered practical or physical options for decision makers. He contrasts this understanding of choice and cost with the subjectivity of opportunity cost in its non-institutional setting. He describes institutional choices as "higher level choices" (Buchanan 2008).

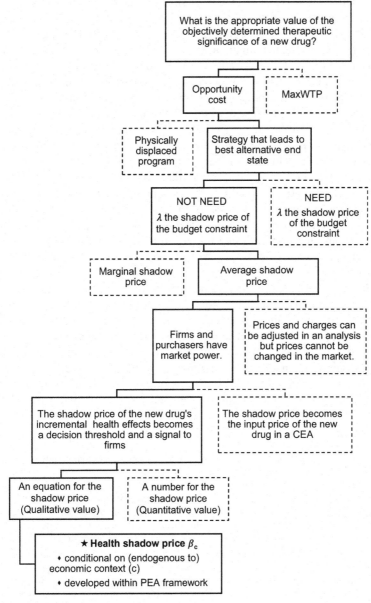

Fig. 6.1 The path to a health shadow price

The Reimburser does not need to know the shadow price of the budget constraint, λ, in order to understand the opportunity cost of reimbursement. In fact it is very likely that this cannot be defined, given the current levels of inefficiency in the health budget. This shadow price should reference the average shadow price of the best alternative input (Kim and Cho 1988). In the context of the reimbursement process, the common reference point across alternative inputs is the amount ΔC, the incremental cost of the new drug at the offer price, the IPER. The opportunity cost of reimbursement is the maximum health effects foregone by allocating ΔC to the reimbursement of the new drug rather than alternative strategies.

Firms, and in some cases the purchaser, have market power; they are price makers not price takers. The patent-owning firm can—and must—select a price for the new drug, unlike the case of a perfectly competitive market for a given drug, where the firm must accept the market price. The Reimburser can use the decision threshold to provide signals to firms, and change this signal if she chooses, as the competitiveness of the market for health inputs changes. The issue of interest is the Reimburser's choice of the decision threshold. The principle suggested by Drummond et al. (2005) is to adjust the input price in a HTA/CEA to reflect its social opportunity cost.[2] This method is not appropriate in this situation; the new drug price problem is about the Reimburser providing a signal about the market for health inputs and the firm using this signal to select an offer price. New drug reimbursement is not an extension of the problem of correcting a charge for an input in a CBA.

Finally, the Reimburser recognises that the initial choice is about the *qualitative* value (an equation) of the threshold, not the *quantitative* value.[3] She notes that there appears to be more certainty regarding the quantitative value of NICE's threshold than its qualitative value.[4] She also recognises that only a qualitative value can be assessed in a theoretical context. Furthermore, a given qualitative value could provide a unique quantitative value for each decision. It is also important to accommodate the possibility that this threshold will be a function of a range of factors, including competition in the market, and hence is likely to vary over time and across decisions.

---

[2] Drummond et al. (2005) provide guidance on how to deal with a non-market price. The authors argue that while there is a theoretical imperative to adjust the "market price" of an input in certain situations, in order to make such an adjustment it was also necessary for health economists to establish a likely benefit to decision making and to use a clear and objective method of making this adjustment. Using the approach suggested by Drummond et al., if there were an acceptable method of adjusting the drug price, the Reimburser could perform a CEA using this adjusted price instead of the firm offer price and then make a decision as to whether the drug was cost-effective. The Reimburser needs to signal the value of the health effects of the new drug to the firm rather than decide of a price of the drug that reflects social opportunity cost.

[3] The *qualitative* value of a decision threshold is its value referenced to an economic, financial or administrative concept such as the shadow price of the budget constraint, the maximum willingness to pay or the aICER of displacement. It is preferable to express it algebraically and with reference to economic theory, for example, the shadow price of the budget constraint. The *quantitative* value of a decision threshold is its numeric value, for example $75,000 per QALY.

[4] The uncertainty in the qualitative value is suggested by Culyer et al. (2007) when the authors refer to potential qualitative values (for example shadow price of the budget constraint or societal willingness to pay) and then go on to that NICE has not specified what it thinks this threshold represents. The relative certainty in its quantitative value (and debate as to whether it should be increased) is indicated by Rafferty (2009) and also Towse(2009).

6.3 PEA, β_c and the Economic Value of Clinical Innovation

In a discussion on the significance of alternative methods of determining the unit cost that should be used in an economic evaluation, when both charges and costs are available, Drummond et al. (2005) conclude that if study results are "relatively insensitive" to choices made about what to identify as the cost of an input then choice of methods only matters if, when studies are compared, differences in these methods are a driver of differences in the final ICER.[5]

PEA reframes how health economists understand the problem of a price for an input, when that input is patented. In PEA it is understood that even if the assessment resulting from a CEA is not sensitive to the way that the unit costs are derived (e.g., charges, or social opportunity cost), the firm's choice of price is sensitive to this choice of method, if the patent holder of this input has market power. If the decision that results from a CEA is not sensitive to the method of costing, and hence price of one of the inputs, then this could be a signal to the owner of this input that the price can be increased without changing the assessment (purchase or not purchase) by the decision maker. That is, even if the drug continues to be assessed as "cost-effective" if the drug "price" is varied in the analysis, (and hence the decision by the purchaser does not vary), the price that a manufacturer will offer will vary as the signal to the firm (the decision threshold) varies.

Furthermore, the maximum acceptable price for the input can be inferred from the value assigned by the Reimburser to health effects via the decision threshold, (as discussed in Part 1 of the dung beetle story). The price assigned to an input either directly (via a unit cost in a HTA/CEA) or indirectly via a decision threshold matters because the patent-holding firm can respond to this signal in ways that impact on both consumer welfare and social welfare. The implications of this strategic context are discussed in detail in Chaps. 8 to 10. In this chapter, a method for determining a reference price, the health shadow price, is presented.

The PEA starting point is to reframe the problem of adjusting the price of an input in a HTA/CEA to reflect the input's social opportunity cost[6] as a problem of:

- Developing a clear, objective and theoretically defensible method;
- Identifying a qualitative value (equation) for the shadow price for the additional health effects of the new drug;
- Referencing against the best alternative strategy; and
- Applying this as a signal (decision threshold) in the reimbursement decision.

---

[5] See page 59 in Drummond et al. (2005).

[6] This approach is nominated by Drummond et al. (2005). It appears to have its origins in Sugden and Williams (1978) and has two problems. The first is that the social opportunity cost appears to be calculated with reference to the maxWTP for the output. The second is that it does not recognise that if the producer has market power, then the price of the input is endogenous to the decision regarding the adoption or otherwise of a program (See example of the dung beetle program).

In this chapter I show that, when used together, the following five concepts provide a clear and objective method of introducing the shadow price into the reimbursement process.

- Opportunity cost as the strategy that leads to the best end-state alternative. This strategy is not the physically displaced strategy (an operational issue) and not necessarily a physical option available to the Reimburser.
- Reimbursement is a strategy comprising two actions: adoption of the new drug and financing of its additional costs.
- PEA is a method whereby the relationship between the price of a new drug and the population's health can be analysed.
- The health shadow price, β_c, is the IPER[7] of a new drug such that the Reimburser:

  - Is indifferent between: the strategy of reimbursing the new drug (adoption and financing); and the best alternative strategy for improving the population's health (which could be improving efficiency).
  - Given: the economic context of the health budget (is it allocatively and technically efficient?); and the optimality with which the additional cost of adoption is financed from the health care budget.

- The economic value of clinical innovation is the clinical value of innovation valued at β_c. This is the appropriate value of the objectively determined therapeutic significance of a new drug, in the context of a market transaction.

6.3.1 The Problem

To illustrate the concepts and define the terminology we initially assume an economically efficient budget *and* perfectly competitive input markets (no market power). These assumptions are relaxed in Chaps. 7 and 8. The nominated strategy (reimbursement) is adoption financed by expansion of the budget (not by displacing existing services). Five parameters need to be defined to derive β_c and hence the shadow price of the new drug in this situation:

1. A maximand (the measure of effect);
2. A nominated strategy and its corresponding effect(s);
3. The constraints that define the set of strategies from which the best alternative strategy will be selected;
4. The set of alternative strategies; and

---

[7] In PEA, the price of a new drug is referred to as an incremental price per additional effect (IPER $=f$). Arithmetically, it is identical to the additional cost per unit effect of the new drug. The term "price" is used instead of the term "cost" to recognise that, unlike the ICER of a QUIT smoking counselling session (for example), the ICER of a new drug is endogenous to the decision to reimburse—it is a price that is up for negotiation.

5. The best alternative strategy from this set.

A simple example of the decision to purchase a new drug and to finance its purchase with the expansion of a budget is used to illustrate these five elements.

1. The *effect or maximand* is health, measured in QALYs.
2. The nominated strategy (R) is reimbursement, which comprises the actions of *adoption* and *financing*.

   (a) *Adoption:* The adoption of a new Drug P is achieved by completely replacing Drug Q with Drug P for target patients. The incremental effect associated with adopting Drug P is $\Delta E^P = 20$ QALYs; the increase in health gains possible for the target patients following the adoption of the new Drug P compared with the best care they would otherwise receive (Drug Q).
   (b) *Financing:* The new drug has an additional financial cost of $\Delta C^P = \$1,000$, which consists entirely of the additional cost of the drug (there are no other financial implications). The additional cost of this new drug is financed by the expansion of the existing health budget by $1,000. The firm's offer price for the new drug, f, is expressed in terms of the IPER[8]:

$$f = \text{IPER} = \frac{\Delta C^P}{\Delta E^P} = \frac{1,000}{20} = \$50 \text{ per QALY.}$$

3. The *constraints* that define the set of alternative strategies (comprising adoption and financing actions) are:

   (a) *The additional financial cost of Drug P ($1,000)*, that is, the alternative adoption action must have an additional financial cost of $1,000 and the financing action, in this case budget expansion, must raise this amount; and
   (b) *The programmes and technologies currently available* to expand or adopt, or to displace to finance any additional cost of the new drug.

4. The *set of alternative strategies* defined by these constraints comprises adoption (or expansion) actions and corresponding financing actions (displacement or budget expansion). The action of adoption (or expansion) of these programmes and technologies must be financed by an amount of $1,000. This set of alternative strategies excludes the mutually exclusive therapies for the group of target patients identified by the nominated strategy, reimbursement of Drug P. The best of the mutually exclusive actions relative to Drug P, Drug Q, is already included in the estimate of the incremental effect of Drug P. The incremental effect of each of the actions and pairs of actions (financing plus adoption is a strategy),

---

[8] The IPER (the incremental price-effectiveness ratio) is used instead of the ICER (the incremental cost-effectiveness ratio) because the additional cost of the new drug to the health system is a function of the price of the new drug, which is in turn the subject of negotiation not the empirical result of a clinical trial.

given the strategies in the constraint set in Step 3, are assumed, in this example, to be known with certainty.

5. The *best alternative strategy* (T) is the strategy from this set of alternative strategies that has the greatest effect. This strategy comprises the adoption action with the greatest effect and the financing option with the minimum reduction in health. In this example there is only one financing option, budget expansion, which never results in displaced health effects. In this example the best alternative strategy is expansion of Programme S with an associated effect, $\Delta E^S = 25$ QALYs and an additional cost of $1,000 that is financed by expansion of the budget.

The reason that Steps (3) and (4) are separated is to allow the economic problem to be changed by either:

- Changing the constraints that defined the set of alternative strategies (for example, there is technological change that expands the number of new programs that could potentially be included, or the methods for financing change); or
- Changes in the alternative strategies (combination of actions) within this set for given constraints (for example, changes in the relative price of inputs).

Both of these types of changes will impact on the incremental cost and effect of alternative strategies, which would be recalculated in Step 4.

6.3.2 Summary Measures

The following summary measures represent the concepts related to β_c and the associated economic value of innovation in the context of a perfectly competitive market and economically efficient health budget. The terminology is expanded for non-optimal initial conditions in Chap. 7.

The Net Health Benefit of Drug P $\Delta E^P (=20 \text{ QALYs})$ is the incremental gain in health for the target patients from using Drug P instead of the best alternative therapy for these patients, Drug Q. In the case of a new drug, it is the effect size, preferably derived from an RCT of the new drug against the best available therapy, multiplied by the number of target patients in the population. It is also referred to as the *clinical value of innovation* (CVI) which emphasises the link between pharmaco-economics (derived from HTA/CEA and the incremental effect) and pharma-economics (which is motivated largely by the economics of pharmaceutical innovation) (See Chap. 4).

The Net Financial Cost of Adopting Drug P $\Delta C^P (=\$1,000)$ is the additional financial cost of the nominated strategy compared with the best alternative therapy (assessed in clinical terms) for that group of patients. These are the additional financial resources that need to be sourced to finance the additional costs of the new drug from the health budget, at the offer IPER. In this example, the financing action is the expansion of the budget.

The Net Health Benefit for the Population of the Strategy of Reimbursement $\Delta E^R (=\Delta E^P = 20$ QALYs) is the net effect on a population's health of reimbursement (adoption and financing). (In contrast, the net effect of the drug ΔE^P is the net effect of adoption for the patient group). In the case of financing by an expanded budget, no existing programme needs to be displaced hence the net health benefit of Strategy R for the population is the same as that of the health effect for target patients from adoption of the new drug. If an existing programme had to be displaced to finance adoption, then the net health effect of reimbursement would be the incremental effect of the new drug less the loss of health effects from displaced services. This issue is explored in Chap. 7.

The Net Health Benefit for the Population of the Best Alternative Strategy T is $\Delta E^T (=\Delta E^S + 0 = 25$ QALYs) Similarly, the net health effect of the best alternative strategy, T, is the same as those of action S (expansion of Program S) because the additional costs are financed by the same action for both reimbursement and the best alternative strategy, namely budget expansion. If T comprised action S financed by the displacement of a second program rather than by budget expansion, the last term would not be "+0" but include the loss to the patients whose program was displaced.

The Net Financial Cost of the Strategy of Reimbursement is $\Delta C^R = \Delta C^P = \Delta C$ where ΔC is the expansion of the budget. If the strategy is financed within a fixed budget the net financial impact of reimbursement on the total budget is 0 even though there is a reallocation of ΔC^P within the health budget. This issue is explored further in Chap. 7.

The Opportunity Cost is expressed as foregone benefit of the nominated strategy, Strategy R (reimbursement, the substitution of Drug Q by Drug P financed by expansion of the budget). It is the effect of the best alternative strategy, T (expansion of Programme S financed by expansion of the budget); 25 QALYs. As stated before, these strategies, R (reimbursement) and T (best alternative), are not mutually exclusive for the group of target patients for the new drug.[9] However, they are mutually exclusive options for the population, where the budget is only expanded to finance one strategy. This opportunity cost is a consequence of the definition of the set of alternative strategies, which in turn defines the opportunity cost in terms of the best alternative use of the fixed budget increment ΔC^P.

The Net Economic Benefit (Health) of the Nominated Strategy (NEBh^R) is Strategy R's impact on the population net the effect of the best alternative strategy, T:

$$\text{NEBh}^R = \Delta E^R - \Delta E^T = 20 - 25 = -5 \text{ QALYs.}$$

---

[9] The mutually exclusive alternative strategy to R for this group of patients is already accommodated in the definition of clinical innovation which is estimated against the best alternative mutually exclusive therapeutic strategy for this patient group.

Hence there is a net economic loss of 5 QALYs as a consequence of reimbursing the new drug at the offer price of f.

The Health Shadow Price β_c is the IPER of the new drug in a specific economic context (c) at which the Reimburser is indifferent between the two strategies of reimbursing the new drug and the best alternative strategy, T.

$$0 = \text{NEBh}^R$$
$$= \Delta E^R - \Delta E^T$$
$$= \frac{\Delta C^P}{f} - \Delta E^T$$
$$= \frac{\$1,000}{f} - 25$$
$$\Rightarrow f = \frac{\$1,000}{25} \text{per QALY}$$
$$\Rightarrow \beta_c = \$40 \text{ per QALY}$$

The (Average) Shadow Price of the Budget Constraint is the maximum gain in health effects as a consequence of budget expansion, without the new drug:

$$\lambda^B = \Delta E^T = \frac{\$1,000}{25} = \$40 \text{ per QALY}.$$

The average shadow price of the budget constraint could also be expressed in terms of units of output (in this case QALYs). This approach is more common in operations research models than health economic models. In this case it would be 25 QALYs.

The Economic Value of Clinical Innovation is $\text{EVCI} = \beta_c \, \Delta E^P = 40 \times 20 = \$800$. This is the economic value of the objectively estimated therapeutic value of the new drug, as estimated for a market where there is competition for alternative ways to produce the health effect.

6.4   Discussion

A number of concepts were introduced in this chapter, some of which are intended to allow distinctions to be drawn between concepts that are currently used interchangeably. Other concepts are unique to PEA. Pairs of concepts are summarised in Table 6.1.

Table 6.1 Summary of PEA concepts

Concept A	Concept B	Distinction
Adoption The clinical decision to substitute therapy A with therapy B or add therapy B to therapy A	Reimbursement The decision to Adopt a new drug and Finance its additional cost from the health budget	Conventionally, the terms adoption and reimbursement are used interchangeably. The characterisation of Reimbursement as two actions, adoption and financing, allows the decision of reimbursement to be related to the net effect on the population (rather than patients) and also allows the optimality of both the adoption and financing actions to be considered separately when defining the health shadow price.
ICER Incremental cost-effectiveness ratio	IPER Incremental price-effectiveness ratio	Arithmetically identical terms. The term IPER is used to distinguish inputs such as new drugs where the price is the subject of negotiation, strategy and market power. The price of the drug is selected by the firm, is not a given and it is not the result of a clinical trial.
ICER As above	aICER (weighted) Average ICER	Typically economists estimate the average ICER for a program and refer to it as the ICER. The term "average ICER" is used to allow for the possibility that if a service is expanded or contracted its aICER will be a function of the direction and the size of the budget change as a consequence of increasing or decreasing marginal costs of the programme.
ΔE^P The net health effect of adopting the new drug	ΔE^R The net effect of reimbursement on the health of the population	The incremental effect of the new drug is its clinical innovation compared to the best existing therapy. The health effect of reimbursement is the net effect of reimbursement on the population. It is a function of the clinical innovation of the drug (adoption) and the method of financing the new drug (displaced services or expanded budget).
$NBh_i = \Delta E^P - \dfrac{\Delta C}{i}$ The conventional net benefit	$NEBh_i = \Delta E^P - \dfrac{\Delta C}{\beta_c}$ The net economic benefit of reimbursement	The conventional net benefit is sometimes referred to as the net economic benefit. It can be valued by a range of values of i including k, n and d. However, strictly speaking, it is only the net economic benefit if it accommodates the economic context, for example, the competition in the market for health inputs and existing inefficiencies. Hence the net economic benefit is the conventional net benefit with β_C as the value of i
λ^B Shadow price of the budget constraint	β_C Shadow price of the health effects of the new drug	In this case, the shadow price of the budget constraint is defined as the maximum additional effect or the additional cost per additional effect, of the expansion of the budget constraint. It is calculated without the new technology β_C is the IPER of the new drug such that, in the specific economic context c, the Reimburser is indifferent between the strategy of reimbursement and the best alternative strategy in terms of their impacts on the population's health.

6.4.1   Key Concepts Expanded

The two key concepts expanded in this section are:

- The net economic benefit measured in health effects; and
- The value of the new drug.

6.4.1.1   The Net Economic Benefit (Health) for the Population

The parameter NEBh^R is the net economic benefit measured in health effects of the strategy of reimbursement. It is an economic value, quantified in health effects, of the precisely defined net health benefit (for the population) of the strategy of reimbursement (adoption and financing). There are a number of ways to express this parameter in the example presented in this chapter, where the economic context is economic efficiency and financing occurs by expanding a budget constraint. In all cases, it is the last term in this equation that gives the NEBh^R its distinctly economic flavour, not monetisation. This term, $-\Delta E^T$ is the foregone benefit to the population of the best alternative strategy for the *population*. For example:

$$\text{NEBh}^R = \Delta E^R - \Delta E^T.$$

However, because the additional costs are financed by budget expansion, there is no net reduction in the health for the population, therefore:

$$\Delta E^R = \Delta E^P.$$

That is, the incremental health gains for the population from reimbursing the new drug are the same as the incremental health effects of the new drug for the target patients. Therefore:

$$\text{NEBh}^R = \Delta E^P - \Delta E^T.$$

The NEBh^R defines the economic value of accessing the clinical innovation from Drug P (ΔE^P) in the context of reimbursement financed by an expanded budget. It defines the economic value in terms of how many additional health gains are available for the population due to reimbursement (ΔE^R), compared with the health effects possible from the best alternative way to use the additional budget funds within existing technologies, ΔE^T.

One way of thinking about this metric is that if there were a gain in the population's health from the new drug when it is adopted and the additional cost were financed by budget expansion, then the benefits to the population from expanding the budget needs to be netted from the benefits of the clinical innovation of the new technology. Hence the economic value of the new drug is the clinical innovation constrained by what could have been achieved with the same additional resources and existing technologies.

6.4.1.2 Value of the New Drug

The *gross effect* of the new drug is E^P, the effect of the drug compared with (constrained by) placebo. *The clinical value of innovation* is the gross effect of the new drug constrained by the opportunity cost of the best alternative therapy for the same patient group. This definition is consistent with the HTA/CEA definition of the clinical innovation of a new therapy:

$$\Delta E^P = E^P - E^Q.$$

The *economic value* of the new drug's clinical innovation is the clinical value of the innovation constrained by the economic context, including factors such as the following, which are discussed further in Chap. 7:

- Whether the budget is fixed or expandable;
- The degree of competition in the market for inputs into health effects;
- Whether or not there is an initial condition of economic efficiency; and
- The optimality or otherwise of displacement if the budget is fixed.

The *health shadow price* β_c is the mechanism by which the economic context is accommodated in the economic value of clinical innovation:

$$\text{EVCI} = \beta_c \Delta E^P.$$

In the example given in this chapter, the EVCI is the gross health benefit of Drug P, E^P, constrained by both E^Q the gross benefit of Drug Q, the best alternative therapeutic strategy for these patients) and ΔE^T (the incremental health gain of the best alternative use of resources, ΔC^P for the population). In the scenarios explored in the following chapters, it is also constrained by the optimality (or otherwise) of the process of displacement. Furthermore, the best alternative strategy is defined by the existing inefficiency in the health care system.

There is an instructive analogue here between the clinical value of innovation and the economic value of clinical innovation.

> The clinician needs information about both the new strategy and the best existing strategy in order to determine the best action for the patient.

By using the clinical value of innovation rather than the gross effect of the new drug, HTA/CEA ensures that we do not attribute the clinical value of innovation of Drug Q, relative to placebo, to Drug P. This technique prevents the adoption of a new drug because it has a clinical advantage compared with placebo when it is less effective than an existing drug. Hence even though patients are better off using the new drug versus no drug, they would be best off using the best existing therapy rather than the new drug.

> The fundholder needs information about the effects of both reimbursement and the best alternative strategy to reimbursement on the population's health to make the best decision for the population.

The economic value of clinical innovation of a new drug is calculated net of the incremental effect of the best alternative strategy to reimbursement. In the case illustrated in this chapter, we need to avoid the situation of attributing the increase in the population's health that is due to the budget expansion to the clinical innovation of the new drug. This technique prevents the following scenario: fundholders expand the budget to finance the new drug and justify this because the health of the population increases. However, if the health of the population would have increased more if the most cost-effective of existing strategies had been adopted, the fundholders have made a suboptimal decision; a different strategy would have resulted in a greater increase in the population's health.

6.5   Conclusion

The Reimburser then reviews her question:

- Is there a shadow price for the health effects of a new drug that:
  - Is based on the opportunity cost of the best alternative way to produce health effects;
  - Can be used as a decision threshold IPER for a new drug; and
  - Is sensitive to the economic context?

PEA is a method whereby the relationship between price of a new drug and the population's health can be analysed. β_c is the IPER of the new drug at which the Reimburser is indifferent between expanding the budget to finance the new drug and financing the best alternative strategy. In the simple example presented in this chapter, where the additional cost of the new drug is financed by budget expansion β_c is no different to the shadow price for the budget constraint, λ. Using β_c as the decision threshold appears no different than using λ. However, the difference (bias and economic loss) between CEA applied with a threshold of λ and PEA with a threshold of β_c arises in the following contexts:

- When there is a fixed or constrained budget and economic inefficiency in that budget; and/or
- When displacement to finance the additional costs of the new drug is suboptimal.

The ways in which β_c accommodates the economic context—and λ fails to do so—are demonstrated in the following chapter.

References

Buchanan J (2008) Opportunity cost. In: Durlauf S, Blume L (eds) The New Palgrave dictionary of economics online, 2nd edn. Palgrave Macmillian, Basingstoke

Culyer A, McCabe C, Briggs A, Claxton K, Buxton M, Akehurst R, Sculpher M, Brazier J (2007) Searching for a threshold, not setting one: the role of the National Institute for Health and Clinical Excellence. J Health Serv Res Policy 12(1):56–58

Drummond MF, Sculpher MJ, Torrance GW et al (2005) Methods for the economic evaluation of health care programmes, 3rd edn. Oxford University Press, Oxford

Kim S, Cho SC (1988) A shadow price in integer programming for management decision. Eur J Oper Res 37(3):328–335

Rafferty J (2009) Should NICE's threshold range for cost per QALY be raised? No. BMJ 338: b185. doi:10.1136/bmj.b185

Sugden R, Williams A (1978) The principles of practical cost-benefit analysis. Oxford University Press, Oxford

Towse A (2009) Should NICEs threshold range for cost per QALY be raised? Yes. BMJ 338:181. doi:10.1136/bmj.b181

Chapter 7
The Health Shadow Price and the Economic Context

Abstract The value of clinical innovation of a new drug is specific to a particular clinical context; the patient group, the clinical protocol and the best alternative therapy. Similarly, the economic value of a given clinical value of innovation is specific to a particular economic context; the financial costs of the proposed and existing therapy, the method of financing the additional costs (budget expansion or displacement of services), the efficiency of the existing allocation and the competition in the market for health inputs. In Chap. 8 the ways in which the health shadow price, β_c and Economic value of clinical innovation, EVCI, capture the economic context of the health budget are illustrated. β_c is derived for four different economic contexts. I show that when the budget is fixed and allocatively inefficient: $\beta_c = (1/n - 1/m + 1/d)^\wedge(-1)$ where n is the average Incremental Cost-Effectiveness, aICER, of the most cost-effective existing technology or programme (in expansion), m is the aICER of the least cost-effective of currently funded technologies or programmes (in contraction) and d is the aICER of the services displaced to finance the additional costs, ΔC^P, of the new drug. The health shadow price is conditional on an economic context, indicated by c. The economic context is defined by factors including the sub-optimality of displacement (m-d), the level of allocative inefficiency in the health budget (m-n), the additional costs that need to be financed (ΔC^P) and the current price structure in the health input market.

7.1 The Reimburser's Problem

The Reimburser understands that β_c is derived within:

- A strategy of reimbursement (adoption and financing);
- An economic context that includes alternative ways to produce health effects; and
- A health budget that may or may not be economically efficient.

© Springer International Publishing Switzerland 2015

B.A.K. Pekarsky, *The New Drug Reimbursement Game*,

DOI 10.1007/978-3-319-08903-4_7

The Reimburser also understands that the best alternative strategy to the strategy of reimbursement of the new technology need not be an actual physical option available to her. Following the definition of opportunity cost from Buchanan (2008) she understands that the best alternative strategy simply needs to represent the alternative resource allocation that maximises the payoff. Hence the choice of the alternative strategy to reimbursement can compensate, at some level at least, the failure of the institution to consider reimbursement of unpatented and unpatentable strategies.

The Reimburser also understands that a threshold IPER for a new drug derived from the health shadow price will accommodate the economic context, for example, the competition in the market to produce health effects. In contrast, a threshold IPER for the drug derived from a maxWTP for health effects will not accommodate the full economic context. However, the Reimburser does not yet understand how the health shadow price accommodates the characteristics of the health budget.

The Reimburser asks two questions.

- How does β_c vary across different reimbursement strategies and economic contexts?
- Why can PEA and not HTA/CEA accommodate the economic context?

The Health Economic Adviser develops four scenarios that illustrate β_c and the EVCI under reimbursement, where adoption is financed in two different ways. The first scenario is an algebraic presentation of the case presented in the previous chapter. The remaining three scenarios illustrate reimbursement under a fixed budget and a range of economic conditions, including allocative inefficiency. These scenarios also illustrate situations of optimal and suboptimal displacement. The nominated strategy in all cases is to reimburse a new drug. The financing of that drug and economic conditions vary across each scenario as summarised in Table 7.1.

> **Note** All analysis and discussion in this book is concerned solely with new drugs that have clinical innovation $\Delta E > 0$ and an additional cost $\Delta C > 0$. The limitations of the ICER under cases where one or both of these conditions is not met are recognised but are not relevant to this discussion. Hence the ICER_i and the conventional net benefit, NB_i are interchangeable as summary metrics of the decision to adopt a new drug.[1]

---

[1] The definitions of ICERi and NBi are presented in the notation glossary and Pekarsky (2012, Appendix 4).

Table 7.1 Four scenarios of economic context

Characteristic	Scenario 1	Scenario 2	Scenario 3	Scenario 4
Adopting a new drug	Yes	Yes	Yes	Yes
Budget	Expandable	Fixed	Fixed	Fixed
How is additional cost of the drug financed?	Expanding budget	Displacing programmes	Displacing programmes	Displacing programmes
Price distortions?	Only new drug	Only new drug	Only new drug	Only new drug
Is current budget efficient?	Economically efficient	Economically efficient	Allocatively inefficient	Technically inefficient
Is displacement optimal? (least cost-effective program displaced)	Not applicable	Optimal or suboptimal	Optimal or suboptimal	Optimal or suboptimal

7.2   Scenario 1: Adoption Financed by Expansion of an Economically Efficient Budget

A Reimburser in a fictional country is *required*[2] to increase the health budget by an amount $\Delta C^P > 0$ and adopt a new drug, P. This requirement to purchase the new drug is a consequence of the new drug being clinically innovative, and in this fictional country, any drug that is clinically innovative must be reimbursed, regardless of the price of that drug. *New drug adoption financed by budget expansion* is the nominated strategy. The budget is currently economically efficient.

The new technology, Drug P, has an offer price expressed as an IPER $f > 0$ and an additional effect compared with the best alternative therapy (clinical value of innovation) for this group of patients of:

$$\text{CVI} = \frac{\Delta C^P}{f} > 0,$$

where $\Delta C^P > 0$ is the additional financial cost of the new drug.

The Reimburser also identifies the most cost-effective (in expansion or adoption)[3] of the existing programmes; Programme N at an aICER of $n > 0$. This is an opportunity to increase the health of the population by an amount:

$$\frac{\Delta C^P}{n} = \Delta E^N > 0,$$

Expansion of Programme N is the best alternative strategy.[4] It is the action with the maximum possible gain that also meets the condition of being financed by expanding the budget constraint by an amount ΔC^P. (See Sect. 6.3.1.) This scenario is illustrated in Fig. 7.1.

---

[2] The "operational" justification is that in this fictional country, the Reimburser is required to adopt the new drug based on consideration of its clinical innovation value only, that is, $\Delta > 0$. From a methodological perspective, this assumption allows us to separate the question of the choice of the decision threshold (explored in Chap. 8 in a game theoretic model) from the question of the economic value of the strategy of reimbursement. It also allows us to exclude the possibility that the firm considers the decision threshold when it sets the price. See also the discussion in the Conclusion to this Chapter.

[3] The program that is the most cost-effective in expansion is defined as follows. The incremental gain in health effect of expanding all existing programs by an amount ΔC^P is estimated. Then the program that gains the largest number of health effects as a consequence of expansion is the most cost-effective program (in expansion). This Program is not necessarily the most cost-effective of all programs. The average cost per effect of the whole program could be more than the cost per effect in expansion if the program has increasing marginal benefit or decreasing marginal cost or both. However there could also be another program or technology that is not yet funded and is only available if the budget is expanded. Hence the best alternative strategy set includes programs and technologies that are either currently funded or not currently funded.

[4] This is Strategy S from Sect. 6.3.

Fig. 7.1 Scenario 1: expandable budget

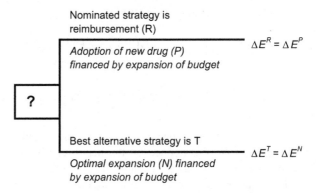

The shadow price (λ) of the budget constraint (B), defined in terms of expansion (e) and measured as an ICER is:

$$\lambda_e^B = \frac{\Delta C^P}{\Delta E^N} = n.$$

This result is the aICER of the additional effects ΔE^N of the most cost-effective programme in expansion, where the additional cost of this programme is financed by expanding the health budget by an amount ΔE^P.

The net financial cost of Strategy R is:

$$\Delta C^P > 0.$$

This is the additional financial cost to the health budget of reimbursing the new drug and it is financed by expansion of the budget.

The net health benefit of Strategy R is:

$$\Delta E^R = \Delta E^P > 0.$$

This is the net health gain to the population as a consequence of reimbursement. This is the same as the gain to the target patients because in this scenario, no services need to be displaced to finance the additional cost of the new drug.

The NEBh of Strategy R (NEBh^R) is:

$$NEBh^R = \Delta E^R - \Delta E^T$$
$$= \Delta E^P - \Delta E^N$$
$$NEBh^R = \Delta C^P \left(\frac{1}{f} - \frac{1}{n} \right). \tag{7.1}$$

This is the gain in health effects for the population as a consequence of Strategy R, ΔE^R, constrained by the health effects, ΔE^T, of the best alternative use of the expanded budget, Strategy T. (See Fig. 7.1).

The health shadow price of the health effects of the new drug is an IPER for the new drug such that the Reimburser is indifferent to the Strategy R and the best alternative strategy, T, that is, the net economic benefit of reimbursement is zero:

$$NEBh^R = 0.$$

Substituting this result in Eq. (7.1) we have:

$$\Delta C^P \left(\frac{1}{f} - \frac{1}{n} \right) = 0$$
$$\Rightarrow \frac{1}{f} = \frac{1}{n}.$$

If $f = n$ then the net economic benefit (health) of reimbursement is 0, therefore the health shadow price is:

$$\beta_c = n.$$

The key parameters derived in this scenario are summarised in Table 7.2 and discussed in Sect. 7.6.

7.3   Scenario 2: Adoption Financed by Displacement in an Economically Efficient Budget

The Reimburser is *required* to adopt a new Drug P, financing its additional cost by displacement of an existing programme. The health budget is fixed and currently economically efficient. The *strategy of reimbursement* (R, the nominated strategy) comprises two actions: displacement followed by adoption. Adoption is financed by displacement of existing programmes rather than expansion of the budget as in Scenario 1. This situation is a consequence of the fixed budget.

The Reimburser does not perform the action of displacement, which is carried out by a separate agency lead by the Displacer, who operates under rules that prevent him from displacing certain types of programmes.[5] Programme D is displaced. It has an aICER of $d > 0$ and hence displacement is at a health loss (or health cost) of:

$$\frac{\Delta C^P}{d} = \Delta E^D.$$

The Reimburser is *required* to use these additional financial resources ΔC^P to finance the additional new drug that has:

- An additional financial cost of $\Delta C^P > 0$;
- An additional effect for the target group of patients $\Delta E^P > 0$; and
- An IPER of:

$$f = \frac{\Delta C^P}{\Delta E^P} > 0.$$

The only criterion for reimbursement that has to be met by the new drug is that $\Delta E^P > 0$ and this new drug meets this criterion. Using PEA, the strategy of reimbursement, R, is understood to comprise the actions of displacement and adoption. It is compared with the best alternative strategy (optimal displacement and optimal expansion) as illustrated in Fig. 7.2. The (non-economic) payoff to reimbursement, R, is the net change in the health of the population.

The Reimburser identifies the least cost-effective (in contraction) of existing programmes; Programme M at an aICER of m. She also identifies the most cost-effective of the existing programmes (in expansion, *given previous contraction*[6]) and programmes and technologies that are not currently funded; this is Programme N at an aICER of n. Therefore the best alternative strategy (T) to the nominated strategy (R) is to displace an amount ΔC^P from the least cost-effective programme (M) at a health effect loss of:

---

[5] The Displacer is not permitted to displace programs that are patented and approved as part of a legally enforceable reimbursement process. He can displace programs that are unpatented and can be contracted by small units, for example a respite care program that can be contracted by reducing the hours of care available by 1 or 100 hours.

[6] How do we identify a program's cost-effectiveness in expansion if there is a fixed budget? First the least cost-effective of existing programs, M needs to be contracted. Then the most cost-effective in expansion of remaining programs is funded. This is the most cost-effective given previous contraction. This device allows for the possibility that the best alternative strategy under a fixed budget has no net health effect if the budget is currently economically efficient.

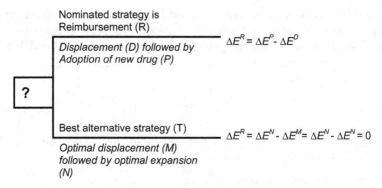

Fig. 7.2 Scenario 2: fixed budget and economic efficiency

$$\frac{\Delta C^P}{m} = \Delta E^M,$$

and use these funds to expand the most cost-effective existing programme (N) at a health gain of:

$$\frac{\Delta C^P}{n} = \Delta E^N.$$

The net health benefit of the best alternative strategy (T) is:

$$\Delta E^T = \Delta E^N - \Delta E^M.$$

The health budget is currently economically efficient and reallocation is assumed to be costless. This implies that after optimal displacement, which is to displace the least cost-effective (in contraction) of existing programmes (M), optimal expansion occurs when the same programme (M) is now refunded because it would then be the most cost-effective (in expansion) of remaining programmes.

If there were another more effective programme that could have been expanded, it would already have been identified because the budget is economically efficient: there is no action that can be performed within existing funds and technologies that would increase the health output.

Hence, at the initial condition of economic efficiency, the net effect of optimal displacement and optimal expansion is zero, $m = n$ and:

$$\Delta E^N = \Delta E^M.$$

Therefore, the best alternative strategy (T) has a net financial cost and net health benefit of zero. This situation is a consequence of the current optimality of allocation ($\Delta E^T = 0$) of a fixed budget ($\Delta C^T = 0$). There is no strategy within current technologies and programmes that can be implemented or expanded to increase the population's health.

The shadow price of the budget (in contraction) is:

$$\lambda_c^B = m(= n).$$

The shadow price of the budget (in expansion given previous contraction (elc) is:

$$\lambda_{e|c}^B = n = m.$$

The nominated strategy of reimbursement (R) comprises two actions: displacement (D) and adoption (P).

The net financial cost of reimbursement is the net financial benefit of displacement and adoption:

$$\Delta C^R = \Delta C^P - \Delta C^D = 0.$$

The net health benefit of Strategy R, ΔE^R is the net effect of adoption and displacement:

$$\Delta E^R = \Delta E^P - \Delta E^D.$$

The NEBh of reimbursement is:

$$\begin{aligned}
\text{NEBh}^R &= \left(\Delta E^P - \Delta E^D\right) - \left(\Delta E^N - \Delta E^M\right) \\
&= \left(\Delta E^P - \Delta E^D\right) - \left(\Delta E^N - \Delta E^N\right) \\
&= \Delta E^P - \Delta E^D - 0 \\
\text{NEBh}^R &= \Delta E^R.
\end{aligned}$$

This is the net heath benefit to the population of reimbursement $\Delta E^P - \Delta E^D$ constrained by the net health benefit for the population of the best alternative use of funds $\Delta E^N - \Delta E^M$. The reason that $\text{NEBh}^R = \Delta E^R$ is that the best alternative strategy to reimbursement in an economically efficient and fixed budget has a net health benefit of zero:

$$\Delta E^T = \Delta E^N - \Delta E^M = \Delta E^N - \Delta E^N = 0.$$

The shadow price of the budget constraint, λ, could be defined in any one of three ways. First, it could be undefined as a result of budget being fixed; there is no point in defining the value of an expanded budget if that budget cannot be expanded and therefore it is not an action in the choice set of alternative strategies. Second, it could be defined as the loss if the budget is contracted,[7] which is in this case m, the aICER of the least cost-effective of the currently funded strategies. Third, it could also be defined as the gain if the budget is expanded by one additional unit. In this case, additional information to that available in the alternative strategy set is required in order to determine the shadow price of the budget constraint. Depending on whether the most cost-effective programme in expansion has increasing or decreasing returns to scale, it could be greater or less than m.

The health shadow price is the IPER of the new drug such that the Reimburser is indifferent between the strategies of R (reimburse) and the best alternative strategy (T, optimal displacement and adoption):

$$NEBh^R = 0$$

$$\Rightarrow \left(\Delta E^P - \Delta E^D\right) - \left(\Delta E^N - \Delta E^M\right) = 0$$

$$\Rightarrow \Delta E^P - \Delta E^D = 0$$

$$\Rightarrow \Delta C^P \left(\frac{1}{f} - \frac{1}{d}\right) = 0.$$

So when $f = d$ the Reimburser is indifferent between the two strategies and hence the quantitative value of shadow price of the health effects from the new drug is d:

$$\beta_c = d.$$

Therefore the economic value of clinical innovation is:

$$EVCI = \beta_c \Delta E^P = d\Delta E^P.$$

The key parameters derived in this scenario are summarised in Table 7.2 and discussed in Sect. 7.6.

7.4 Scenario 3: Adoption Financed by Displacement in an Economically Inefficient Budget

As presented in Table 7.1, Scenario 3 has only one difference to Scenario 2: the initial condition in the health budget is allocative inefficiency rather than economic efficiency. The nominated strategy is reimbursement of Drug P: adoption of the new drug financed by displacement of an existing programme. Consider the set of alternative strategies identified in Step 4 in Chap. 6. This set contains many actions

---

[7] The shadow price when the budget is contracted by one unit is consistent with the operations research use of the term and when it is expanded, the economic use (See Sect. 5.3.1).

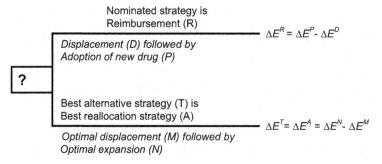

Fig. 7.3 Scenario 3 fixed budget and allocative inefficiency

that are displacement and many actions that are adoption or expansion. It can be considered as the set from which the set of possible options identified in programme budgeting marginal analysis (PBMA) is drawn.[8]

As represented in Fig. 7.3, the best alternative strategy (T) is optimal reallocation (A) of ΔC^P from Programme M (the least cost-effective program in contraction) to Programme Program N (the most cost-effective in expansion, conditional on previous contraction) where $n = m$. Optimal reallocation comprises two actions from the set of alternative actions—contraction of Program M (financing) and expansion of Program N (adopting).[9]

Therefore, as a consequence of existing allocative *inefficiency*:

$$\Delta E^T = \Delta E^A = \Delta E^N - \Delta E^M > 0.$$

Note The distinction between ΔE^T and ΔE^A is that the former is the outcome of the best strategy, T, from the set of alternative strategies whereas the latter is the best of strategy a particular type of strategy (reallocation) from this set of alternative strategies. The best alternative reallocation strategy is always reallocation from Programme M to Programme N. However, if another type of strategy such as the investment in changed practice is included in this set then the best alternative strategy, T, from this set could change. [See Scenario 4, summarised in this chapter in Sect. 7.5 and reported in full in Pekarsky (2012, Appendix 5)].

---

[8] PBMA has a long history and its preeminent advocate in Health Economics is the late Professor Gavin Mooney. The first text I read on this topic was "Choices for health care: a practical introduction to the economics of health provision." (Mooney et al. 1986) I have also been fortunate enough to observe Gavin take a group through the process of PBMA. The set of all alternative actions in Step (4) of PEA is essentially a formalised version of identifying activity at the margin in PBMA.

[9] Why is Strategy A, optimal reallocation, described as the best alternative strategy, T? Shouldn't the two actions of optimal displacement and adoption each be described as the best alternative? The important point is that pairs of displacement and adoption in such a set are about the strategy to reallocate, which, like the term reimbursement, describes two actions. Reimbursement is a qualitatively different strategy to the strategies of (1) Reallocation, and (2) budget expansion and new Program adoption.

The net financial cost of Strategy R is $\Delta C^P - \Delta C^P = 0$ and therefore the net financial cost of the best alternative strategy is also zero. This is because the budget is fixed and therefore there is no net financial cost of either strategy. This is the case even though $\Delta C^P > 0$, that is the net cost of adoption is greater than zero.

The net health benefit for the population of Strategy R is $\Delta E^P - \Delta E^D$ and the impact of the best alternative strategy to R (reallocation, Strategy A, which is optimal adoption and optimal displacement) is $\Delta E^N - \Delta E^M$.

The NEBh for Strategy R is:

$$\text{NEBh}^R = \Delta E^R - \Delta E^T$$
$$= \left(\Delta E^P - \Delta E^D \right) - \left(\Delta E^N - \Delta E^M \right)$$
$$= \left(\frac{\Delta C^P}{f} - \frac{\Delta C^P}{d} \right) - \left(\frac{\Delta C^P}{n} - \frac{\Delta C^P}{m} \right) \qquad (7.2)$$
$$\text{NEBh}^R = \Delta C^P \left(\frac{1}{f} - \frac{1}{d} - \frac{1}{n} + \frac{1}{m} \right).$$

The health shadow price is the IPER of the new drug at which the net economic benefit of Strategy R is zero, that is, where the Reimburser is indifferent between reimbursement and the strategy of optimal reallocation. Using Eq. (7.2):

$$\text{NEBh}^R = 0$$
$$= \left(\frac{1}{f} - \frac{1}{d} - \frac{1}{n} + \frac{1}{m} \right)$$
$$\Rightarrow f = \left(\frac{1}{n} - \frac{1}{m} + \frac{1}{d} \right)^{-1}$$
$$\Rightarrow \beta_c^\alpha = \left(\frac{1}{n} - \frac{1}{m} + \frac{1}{d} \right)^{-1},$$

where the superscript α refers to this particular health shadow price as relating to the best alternative reallocations across existing programmes. (In the following section, a set of alternative strategies that includes only investment strategies is used.)

The economic value of clinical innovation is the clinical value of innovation valued by its health shadow price.

$$\text{EVCI} = \beta_c^\alpha \Delta E^P = \left(\frac{1}{n} - \frac{1}{m} + \frac{1}{d}\right)^{-1} \Delta E^P.$$

The key parameters derived in this scenario are summarised in Table 7.2 and discussed in Sect. 7.6.

7.5 Scenario 4: Adoption Financed by Displacement in an Economically Inefficient Budget (Investment Version)

Scenario 4 is presented in detail in Pekarsky (2012, Appendix 5). The key parameters derived in this scenario are summarised in Table 7.2. In summary, Scenario 4 demonstrates that if there is an option to invest ΔC^P today in changed practice that will reduce the aICER of a programme in the future, then there is a parameter that can capture both the reduction in static efficiency today (for 1 year taking ΔC^P away from the least cost-effective programme) as well as the gain in dynamic efficacy that occurs because the future aICER of the programme is lower than the current aICER. That parameter is μ. The superscript v on the health shadow price β_c allows the distinction to be drawn between the health shadow price derived from investment strategies β_c^v and the health shadow price derived from reallocation strategies, β_c^a.

7.6 Results

The variation in both β_c and ECVI, across the four scenarios is presented in Table 7.2. The properties of these parameters are then discussed.

7.6.1 Properties of Parameters

We assume that all of the following parameters are greater than zero: $f, m, d, n, \Delta E^P$ and ΔC^P. We also continue to assume that the Reimburser in this fictional country must reimburse the new drug, regardless of the offer price (IPER) of f, provided that new drug meets the condition that $\Delta E^P > 0$.

What are the properties of the parameters ΔE^P, ΔC^P, ΔE^R, λ^B, β_c and EVCI ($= \beta_c \Delta E^P$) as illustrated by the four scenarios?

The Clinical Innovation of the New Drug ΔE^P The clinical innovation of the new drug ΔE^P is constant across these scenarios. The drivers of the value of clinical innovation of a given drug are not specified in this chapter. They include the choice of comparator, the clinical protocol, the duration of therapy and the dose. These determinants of ΔE^P are accommodated by HTA/CEA methods. (See Chap. 4)

The Additional Financial Cost of Adoption to the Health Budget $\Delta C^P (= f \Delta E^P)$
The additional financial cost to the health budget (i.e. the amount that must be financed), ΔC^P is constant across these scenarios. The drivers of change in ΔC^P include all those factors that determine ΔE^P. The additional driver is the price (or unit costs) of resources such as diagnostic tests and the IPER of the new drug. In Chap. 8, the consequences of recognising that f and hence ΔC^P is a function of the Reimburser's maximum acceptable IPER (decision threshold) are explored.

The Conventional Net Benefit NB$_i$ The conventional net benefit value remains constant regardless of the economic context and varies with the administrative choice of i, (the decision threshold) which, in Table 7.2 is k.

The Net Effect of Reimbursement on the Population's Health ΔE^R is less than zero when: (1) the budget is fixed and (2) the aICER of displaced services is less than the IPER for the new drug. The net effect of reimbursement on the population's health is a function of d and f. $\Delta E^R{}_{max}$ for a fixed budget, given the requirement to reimburse the new drug at the price f occurs when d is maximised, that is, displacement is optimal when d is maximised and hence $d = m$.

The Net Economic Benefit of Reimbursement (Health) NEBh^R Assuming that adoption is a requirement, then the NEBh^R is maximised when: (1) the health benefits of the new drug are greater than those of the best alternative strategy (adoption is optimal, $f < n$) and (2) displacement is optimal ($d = m$). The conditions under which the NEBh^R is positive are characterised and the limitations of alternative thresholds to the health shadow price are demonstrated in the three inequalities detailed below.

- Inequality One: Net Effect of Reimbursement vs. Improved Economic Efficiency.

$$\text{NEBh}^R > 0.$$

Now referring to Eq. (7.2):

$$\Rightarrow \Delta C^P \left(\left(\frac{1}{f} - \frac{1}{d} \right) - \left(\frac{1}{n} - \frac{1}{m} \right) \right) > 0$$

$$\Rightarrow \left(\frac{1}{f} - \frac{1}{d} \right) - \left(\frac{1}{n} - \frac{1}{m} \right) > 0 \qquad (7.3)$$

$$\Rightarrow \left(\frac{1}{f} - \frac{1}{d} \right) > \left(\frac{1}{n} - \frac{1}{m} \right).$$

This inequality identifies the conditions under which the NEBh^R is positive by comparing the strategies of reimbursement (on the left) and reallocation to reduce economic inefficiency (on the right). From Eq. (7.2), we observe that the NEBh^R can be negative even if the net effect of displacement and adoption is positive ($\Delta E^R > 0$). This occurs if there is sufficient allocative inefficiency ($m > n$) to offset the gain target patients due to the adoption of the new drug, hence generating a net economic loss—the strategy of reallocation would have resulted in more health gains for the population.

Under the use of d as the decision threshold (CEA$_d$), the Reimburser would only adopt the new drug if $f \leq d$. The net health benefit of reimbursement (ΔE^R) is never negative in this case, however, the NEBh^R will be negative even if the $\Delta E^R > 0$ if the best alternative strategy (optimal adoption and displacement) is more effective than reimbursement. Thus even though the $\Delta E^R > 0$ under CEA$_d$, ΔE^R is not necessarily maximised.

If we use the aICER of the most cost-effective of alternative strategies as the decision threshold, then we would adopt if $n \geq f$. In this case, the net benefit for the population will always be positive or equal to zero, because the aICER of the program that is displaced can never be more than the most cost-effective of existing programs in expansion ($n \leq d \leq m$). Hence, because $n \geq f$ and $d \geq n$, then $d \geq f$ and the net effect of displacement and adoption is always positive. However, if displacement is suboptimal ($m > d$) then there would be a net economic loss to reimbursement under n as a threshold, regardless of the net impact on the population.

- Inequality two: optimality of adoption vs. optimality of displacement

  Rearranging Eq. (7.3) we have:

  $$\left(\frac{1}{f} - \frac{1}{n}\right) > \left(\frac{1}{d} - \frac{1}{m}\right). \tag{7.4}$$

This inequality identifies the conditions under which the NEBh^R is positive by comparing the degree of optimality of adoption (left side of equation) with that of the optimality of displacement (right side). If displacement is suboptimal ($d \leq m$), the net economic benefit could still be positive, but not maximised, provided that adoption is optimal ($f \leq n$). However, the reverse is not the case. If adoption is suboptimal then there will always be a net economic loss, because $d \leq f$.

- Inequality three: price of new drug vs. health shadow price

  Rearranging Eq. (7.4) we have:

  $$\frac{1}{f} > \left(\frac{1}{n} + \frac{1}{d} - \frac{1}{m}\right) = \frac{1}{\beta_c} \tag{7.5}$$

  $$\Rightarrow \beta_c > f.$$

By definition, if the IPER of the new drug is β_c then the Reimburser is indifferent between Strategy R (reimbursement) and the best alternative strategy. Therefore, only under the health shadow price as the decision threshold is the NEBh^R never less than zero and hence the health of the population maximised.

The Shadow Price of the Budget Constraint λ^B   The shadow price of the budget constraint is defined when the budget is constrained and economically efficient; it is the aICER of the most cost-effective program in expansion, n. When the budget is fixed and economically inefficient, λ^B could be defined using the operations research definition, the minimum loss under budget contraction, which in this case is the least cost-effective programme in contraction with an aICER of m. Alternatively, it could be undefined.

The Health Shadow Price β_c   The only case where β_c could be greater than n is when the health budget is fixed and economically efficient (Scenario 2). In this case, the opportunity cost of Strategy R is zero, and β_c is the aICER of the displaced programme. If there is a constrained budget and existing economy efficiency (Scenario 1), β_c is n. If there is fixed budget and allocative or technical inefficiency (Scenarios 3 and 4), then $\beta_{c\ max}$ is n.

Proof by contradiction is as follows:
If:

$$\beta_c > n \Rightarrow \frac{1}{n} > \frac{1}{\beta_c}$$

$$\Rightarrow \frac{1}{n} > \left(\frac{1}{n} - \frac{1}{m} + \frac{1}{d} \right)$$

$$\Rightarrow \frac{1}{m} > \frac{1}{d}$$

$$\Rightarrow d > m.$$

However, M is the least cost-effective of all programmes in contraction and d is the aICER of the displaced services (a contracted programme) therefore $m \geq d\ \forall m$, d. Therefore $\beta_{c\ max}$ is n. If there is allocative inefficiency and a fixed budget then β_c is maximised when displacement is optimal ($d = m$).

The Economic Value of the New Drug's Clinical Innovation, EVCI   The economic value of the new drug's clinical innovation, $EVCI = \beta_c \Delta E^P$, varies across scenarios. As the competition from other ways of generating health effects increases, the economic value of the clinical innovation decreases. As the suboptimality of displacement decreases ($d \to n$), so does the economic value of Strategy R and hence the economic value (market price) of the new drug.

7.7 Discussion

What advantages does PEA offer over HTA/CEA? What are the differences between the two methods? PEA does not replace HTA/CEA, which estimates the consequences of the adoption decision, ΔE^P and ΔC^P.

- PEA identifies the strategy of reimbursement (adoption and financing) whereas HTA/CEA identifies the action of adoption.
- PEA quantifies the net health effect for the population of the reimbursement decision, whereas HTA/CEA quantifies the net health effect for target patients from the adoption decision.
- PEA identifies whether there is an alternative strategy that is preferable to reimbursement whereas HTA/CEA only compares the actions of adopt or not adopt.
- β_c is endogenous to the reimbursement decision (it captures suboptimality of displacement) and to the economic context (it captures the best alternative strategy including the strategy of improving inefficiency, technical or allocative).
- PEA appropriately attributes an increase in the population's health following reimbursement to clinical innovation, rather than the strategies of increasing the budget or improving existing inefficiency. The $NEBh^R$ is always estimated net of the best alternative strategy.

7.7.1 The Reimburser's Questions

- How does β_c vary across different reimbursement strategies and economic contexts?

  The economic context of reimbursement varies as a consequence of the method of financing (budget expansion or displacement),); the optimality of displacement, the availability of alternative strategies to improve the health outcomes of the budget, and existing inefficiency in the health budget. This is analogous to the net health benefit of adoption of a new drug for a patient group (its clinical innovation) varying as a consequence of the patient group, duration and dose of therapy, patient compliance with therapy, position of therapy in the clinical context (first-, second- or third-line) and the best available alternative strategy available for that patient group.

Unlike the maxWTP for the health effects of the new drug, β_c captures this variation in economic context; it is endogenous to the economic context. This occurs for the following reasons:

- β_c is solved by finding the IPER of the health effects of the new drug at which the Reimburser is indifferent between the reimbursement of the new drug and the best available alternative strategy, which can be the strategy of reducing inefficiency;

- The difference in the net health effects of the two strategies captures the economic context of inefficiency and whether the budget is fixed or constrained; and
- If the optimality of displacement varies, so will the net health effect of reimbursement.

The maxWTP for given health effects from a new drug does not capture this information; it is constant across all economic contexts. This is analogous to the clinical effect of the new drug (P) being constant, if it were derived from a comparison with placebo, regardless of the changes in the best available therapy.

If we change the set of alternative strategies from which the best alternative strategy is selected, we change β_c. This is demonstrated with the introduction of the opportunities for investment. This is analogous to the change in ΔE and ΔC if the comparator is the best alternative pharmacotherapy vs. a comparator of the best alternative non-pharmacotherapy (e.g. surgery or physiotherapy). The change in alternative strategy could also be consistent with an alternative maximand or set of maximands, an issue explored further in the Conclusion to this book.

- Why can PEA and not HTA/CEA accommodate the economic context?

    The key mechanism of PEA is its definition of the strategy of reimbursement (as adoption and displacement) which in turn accommodates: (1) payoff to the population rather than target patients; and (2) the inefficiency in the health budget and in displacement.

    The first way that PEA accommodates the economic context is by defining the nominated strategy as reimbursement, which comprises the two actions of adoption and displacement. In this way the payoff of the strategy of reimbursement in a fixed budget is the net effect of the health effects to the population of adoption and displacement. This is in contrast to conventional HTA/CEA decision analytic structures, which define the nominated strategy as adoption; typically substitution of the best available drug with the new drug. In such a model, the payoff to the strategy of adoption is the additional cost and effect of the new drug compared with the best existing therapy. The payoff in HTA/CEA is to the target patients and not the overall population. In PEA the payoff of the additional effect for the target patient is accommodated as the health payoff to adoption but this payoff is netted by the loss to the population as a consequence of displacement.

    The second way that PEA accommodates the economic context is by defining the best alternative strategy as comprising the best alternative actions to displacement and adoption in the Reimbursement strategy. This method allows for issues such as inefficiency in displacement (suboptimal displacement) and inefficiency in the health budget to be accommodated in the net economic benefit of reimbursement.

7.8 Conclusion

In summary, β_c is the IPER at which the Reimburser is indifferent between reimbursing the new drug (adoption to place drug in a clinical context plus displacement to finance its additional costs) and the best alternative strategy, given the economic conditions and sub-optimality of displacement. This is the IPER of the new drug at which the net economic benefit to the population of the strategy of reimbursement is zero. β_c is endogenous to the reimbursement decision and is defined by: (1) the incremental cost and effect of the new drug; (2) the economic context (health sector inefficiency and type of budget constraint); and (3) the optimality of displacement. It is the choice of decision threshold that will ensure that the net economic benefit is never negative.

The assumption that the Reimburser must reimburse the new drug regardless of the price is clearly unrealistic. Primarily, it is a device to identify the net effect of the strategy of reimbursement (adoption and displacement) at a given price and decision threshold. If the strategy of reimbursing the new drug has a positive net economic benefit (health) then reimbursement is population health-maximising compared with the best alternative strategy, where these alternatives include strategies to reduce existing inefficiency, both allocative and technical.

A second advantage of using the device (forced reimbursement) is that by assuming that the Reimburser must reimburse the new drug, regardless of the price, we do not need to consider the way that the firm chooses a price. In particular, we do not need to consider whether the IPER is exogenous or endogenous to the decision process. In Chap. 8, I show why it is more realistic to assume that the price of the new drug is endogenous, rather than exogenous, to the reimbursement process. The choice by the firm of the price of the new drug is a function of the choice of decision threshold; the higher the decision threshold, the higher the firm's offer price. Price is a strategic decision by the firm, which considers the likely response by the institution when it prices the new drug.

The strategic element of new drug reimbursement was suggested in Chap. 5. It is the behaviour of the monopolist bike shop owner who does not put price tags on her bikes and instead waits for the purchaser to his maxWTP. It is the action of the dung beetle patent holder who waits until the maxWTP is revealed by the Council to present the price of the dung beetle. It is also the reason why it is not sufficient to simply find a shadow price of the new drug, use it as an input in a HTA/CEA and make the reimbursement decision on the basis of a shadow price adjusted ICER. The economic value of the new drug is signalled via the decision threshold to firms which will consider this information when they select their offer price. The opportunity for firms to act strategically when they price new drugs is one of the reasons why the problem set up in Drummond et al. (2005) needed to be reframed for PEA in Chap. 6. The firm is a player—it chooses the offer price.

Chapter 8, which is about the high stakes game of drug reimbursement, introduces three additional features of PEA that further distinguish it from HTA/CEA:

Table 7.2 Comparison of the value of the key parameters under the four scenarios of economic context

Parameter	Scenario 1: economic efficiency and financed by budget expansion	Scenario 2: economic efficiency and financed by displacement	Scenario 3: allocative inefficiency and financed by displacement	Scenario 4: technical inefficiency and financed by displacement
Clinical value of innovation (target patients) ΔE^P	$CVI = \Delta E^P$	$CVI = \Delta E^P$	$CVI = \Delta E^P$	$CVI = \Delta E^P$
Net health effects from reimbursement (population) ΔE^R	$\Delta E^R = \Delta E^P - 0 = \Delta E^P$	$\Delta E^R = \Delta E^P - \Delta E^D$	$\Delta E^R = \Delta E^P - \Delta E^D$	$\Delta E^R = \Delta E^P - \Delta E^D$
Conventional Net Benefit NB (k)	$NB_k = k\Delta E^P - \Delta C^P$	$NB_k = k\Delta E^P - \Delta C^P$	$NB_k = k\Delta E^P - \Delta C^P$	$NB_k = k\Delta E^P - \Delta C^P$
Net economic benefit from reimbursement (health) $NEBh^R$	$NEBh^R = \Delta E^R - \Delta E^N$	$NEBh^R = \Delta E^R - 0$ $= \Delta E^P - \Delta E^D$ $= \Delta C^P \left(\dfrac{1}{f} - \dfrac{1}{d}\right)$	$NEBh^R = (\Delta E^P - \Delta E^D) - (\Delta E^N - \Delta E^M)$ $= \Delta C^P \left(\left(\dfrac{1}{f} - \dfrac{1}{d}\right) - \left(\dfrac{1}{n} - \dfrac{1}{m}\right)\right)$	$NEBh^R = (\Delta E^P - \Delta E^D) - (\varphi\Delta E^G - \Delta E^M)$ $= \Delta C^P \left(\left(\dfrac{1}{f} - \dfrac{1}{d}\right) - \left(\dfrac{1}{\mu} - \dfrac{1}{m}\right)\right)$
Net financial cost of adoption (target patients) ΔC^P	ΔC^P	ΔC^P	ΔC^P	ΔC^P

	$\Delta C^R = \Delta C^P$	$\Delta C^P - \Delta C^P = 0$	$\Delta C^P - \Delta C^P = 0$	$\Delta C^P - \Delta C^P = 0$
Net financial effect of reimbursement (Population) ΔC^R				
Health shadow price β_c	$\beta_c = n$	$\beta_c = d$	$\beta_c = \left(\frac{1}{n} - \frac{1}{m} + \frac{1}{d}\right)^{-1}$	$\beta_c = \left(\frac{1}{\mu} - \frac{1}{m} + \frac{1}{d}\right)^{-1}$
Shadow price of the budget in expansion λ_e^B	$\lambda_e^B = n$	Unknown/not defined	Unknown/not defined	Unknown/not defined
Shadow price of the budget in expansion conditional on initial contraction $\lambda_{e|c}^B$	n/a	$\lambda_{e|c}^B = n = m$	Unknown	Unknown
Economic value of clinical innovation EVCI	$EVCI = n\Delta E^P$	$EVCI = d\Delta E^P$	$EVCI = \left(\frac{1}{n} - \frac{1}{m} + \frac{1}{d}\right)^{-1} \Delta E^P$	$EVCI = \left(\frac{1}{\mu} - \frac{1}{m} + \frac{1}{d}\right)^{-1} \Delta E^P$

d is the aICER of the services displaced to finance the additional cost of the new drug

m is the aICER of the least cost-effective service in contraction

n is the aICER of the most cost-effective service in expansion

μ is the parameter that captures the gain in health effects for one program by investing in improved practice in terms of an aICER

φ is the parameter that captures the net present value of additional health effects possible from changed practice in Program G

- The Reimburser considers net economic benefit (health) when she makes the reimbursement decision, hence taking into account the economic context;
- A firm uses its market power to select the price of the new drug; and
- Game theoretic rather than decision theoretic models are used to accommodate this strategic (rather than price-taking) behaviour by firms.

References

Buchanan J (2008) Opportunity cost. In: Durlauf S, Blume L (eds) The New Palgrave dictionary of economics online, 2nd edn. Palgrave Macmillian, Basingstoke

Mooney G, Russell E, Weit R (1986) Choices for health care: a practical introduction to the economics of health provision, 2nd edn, Studies in social policy. Macmillan, London

Pekarsky BAK (2012) Trust, constraints and the counterfactual: reframing the political economy of new drug price. Dissertation, University of Adelaide. http://digital.library.adelaide.edu.au/dspace/handle/2440/79171. Accessed 25 Dec 2013

Chapter 8
The "New Drug Reimbursement" Game

Abstract If a new drug's incremental price-effectiveness ratio (IPER) is above the health shadow price, β_c, the best alternative strategy to new drug reimbursement will result in more health benefits to the population, for the same financial cost. The historic decision threshold (k) in most countries is likely to be significantly higher that the health shadow price. If a regulator chooses to reject a new drug as a consequence of adopting the lower threshold, firms might make the following threat: At IPERs below k, it will not be financially viable to supply most new drugs to this country. The weight of this threat could be significant, particularly when the new drugs have substantial clinical benefit for some patient groups. How should a rational institution respond? In this chapter, this question is first analysed in a conventional decision theoretic (non-strategic) model as the optimal response by regulators to historic evidence of the price of new drugs. Then the question is analysed within a price-effectiveness analysis (PEA) framework. PEA uses an applied game theoretic model that assumes firms act strategically and that the health of the population, not the target patients, is the maximand. I conclude that the decision to reimburse a new drug is best analysed as a game with multiple players who act strategically and where the objective of the Institution is to maximise the population's health. The second conclusion is that the population health-maximising response to the threat is to maintain a threshold price of β_c.

8.1 The Reimburser's Problem

The Reimburser announces that she will pay no more than β_c for the additional health effects from new drugs. She estimates β_c to be in the order of $5,042 per additional QALY at this time[1]; only 6.7 % of the max WTP for an additional QALY

---

[1] This hypothetical value was derived as follows. The most cost-effective of existing programs (n) is a dental program with a aICER in expansion of $7,500 per QALY. The least cost-effective of current programs in contraction is a screening program with an ICER of $110,000 per QALY. The program most likely to be replaced is a respite care program with an aICER of $13,500. The value of $\beta_c = \left(\frac{1}{7,500} + \frac{1}{13,500} - \frac{1}{110,000} \right)^{-1} = \$5,042$.

© Springer International Publishing Switzerland 2015
B.A.K. Pekarsky, *The New Drug Reimbursement Game*,
DOI 10.1007/978-3-319-08903-4_8

of \$75,000, which is the prevailing maximum acceptable IPER. A group of clinicians approaches the Reimburser with evidence that the majority of the new innovative drugs over the last 10 years were priced at the historic threshold of k (Devlin and Parkin 2004). These clinicians also refer to an excerpt from an article in *The New York Times* that suggests that society can expect to continue to pay high IPERs for new effective drugs into the future.

> Until now, drug makers have typically defended high prices by noting the cost of developing new medicines. But executives at Genentech and its majority owner, Roche, are now using a separate argument—citing the inherent value of life-sustaining therapies. If society wants the benefits, they say, it must be ready to spend more for treatments like Avastin and another of the company's cancer drugs, Herceptin, which sells for \$40,000 a year. "As we look at Avastin and Herceptin pricing, right now the health economics hold up, and therefore I don't see any reason to be touching them," said William M. Burns, the chief executive of Roche's pharmaceutical division and a member of Genentech's board. "The pressure on society to use strong and good products is there." (Berenson 2006)

The clinicians argue that these historic and future prices are solid evidence that if the maximum acceptable IPER were lowered, many of the future drugs with significant clinical value of innovation and very high costs would not be available to patients because they would not be reimbursed. Patients will be worse off as a result. The evidence that new drugs tend to be priced at the decision threshold is consistent with the Reimburser's experience; most new drugs reimbursed in the last 10 years had an IPER substantially above β_c and close to the max WTP. Given this evidence of the historic IPER of new drugs, the Reimburser is unsure whether she should enforce β_c as the threshold IPER.

The Reimburser asks her Health Economic Adviser two questions:

- Will this lower maximum IPER mean that drugs that would otherwise have been reimbursed at prices above \$5,042 per QALY will no longer be available to the population at a subsidised price?
- If fewer new drugs are available as a consequence of a lowered maximum IPER, will this make the population worse off than it would have been under the existing maximum IPER of \$75,000?

The Health Economic Adviser suggests one more question:

- How should the rational Institution respond to the following threat:

   - If the threshold is reduced to β_c, less than 15 % of the new drugs that would otherwise be approved will be made available to patients. The population will be worse off as a consequence of a lower threshold price.

8.2   A Decision Theoretic Model of the Clinicians' Case

The problem posed by the clinicians can be represented as a DTM with the following structure: the assumptions, strategies and payoffs that will lead to the prediction that the number of NMEs that are reimbursed will reduce if the threshold IPER reduces.

Such a view of the world is represented in Fig. 8.1 for the (hypothetical) case of the evidence from the previous year of 24 new drug reimbursements, where these new drugs had a proven clinical innovation compared with the best alternative therapy. The (hypothetical) evidence shows that of the 24 NMEs reimbursed in the previous year, only two had an IPER at or below $\beta_c = \$5,042$ per QALY. The clinicians argue that this evidence suggests that only two of the NMEs reimbursed in the previous year would have been subsidised at the maximum acceptable IPER of β_c. This situation would represent a loss of 22 NMEs at an average effect of $\Delta \hat{E}^p$ per NME, and hence a loss these patients health effects of $22 \ \Delta \hat{E}^p$. The clinicians produce further evidence that suggests that the average value of $\Delta \hat{E}^p$ was 850 QALYs per year in the year the drugs were reimbursed.[2] Therefore, if these drugs had not been available, around 18,700 QALYs per year in benefits to these patients would not have been experienced.

The world within which this DTM resides is supported, implicitly, by three key assumptions.

1. The budget is assumed to expand to accommodate any purchase at or below the threshold acceptable IPER; it is not fixed and there is no requirement to displace any services to finance the new drug. This is an unconstrained budget in PEA terminology. (See Sect. 3.3)
2. The payoff to reimbursement is the increase in the health of the target patient group $\Delta \hat{E}^p$. Therefore, given that there is no displacement and no unfunded "value for money" option (the budget is unconstrained), we can conclude that the population will be worse off by an amount $22\Delta \hat{E}^p$ if fewer clinically innovative future drugs are funded than would otherwise be the case.
3. There is no other price below the offer price at which these firms could produce and sell the drug, that is, there is no lower price where $\pi \geq 0$ (where π is the firm's economic rent).

These three assumptions lead to a position that is summarised as follows:

---

[2] This estimate would be difficult to derive in practice. It could be derived by multiplying the average incremental QALY gain per patient (derived when the ICER is calculated) by the number of patients who *commence* a course of treatment each year and calculated for the expected duration of their treatment and benefits. In following years, it would be necessary to ensure that the continuing patients whose benefits were included as a future benefit for patients commencing in previous years are not double (triple, quadruple…) counted.

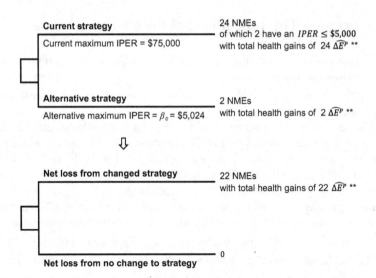

Fig. 8.1 The loss in health due to lowered price: a decision analytic perspective

1. No firms will change their offer price as a response to a change in the threshold IPER signalled by the Reimburser;
2. A reduced threshold IPER will lead to a reduction in the number of NMEs approved by the Reimburser; and
3. As a consequence, under a lower threshold, the population will be worse off than would otherwise be the case.

The three assumptions that premise the above position are not necessarily applicable to the economic context of reimbursement. First, not all health budgets can be expanded to accommodate all purchases that are below an exogenously-determined threshold IPER. This assumption could be appropriate in some jurisdictions but not in the country of interest. Second, the payoff of an additional NME to target patients is $\Delta \hat{E}^p$, but the net impact on the population's health as a consequence of the strategy of Rin a fixed budget is $\Delta \hat{E}^p - \Delta \hat{E}^D$, where $\Delta \hat{E}^D$ is the average health effects displaced to finance the additional costs of a new drug. There could be a loss in potential health gains $\Delta \hat{E}^p$ to target patients if a drug that would otherwise be reimbursed is not subsidised. However, the services that would otherwise have been displaced to finance the new drug are no longer displaced. Therefore the reduction in health gains to the target patients would need to be offset by the gain $\Delta \hat{E}^D$ to patients whose services are not displaced. Third, if firms have market power, their current offer price is *not necessarily* the lowest price at which they would be prepared to produce and sell the drug. Firms with market power can price above the marginal cost of production because there is a lack of competition from other firms willing to increase market share by offering a lower price.[3]

The applied economic model developed in the following section accommodates the three characteristics described in the previous paragraph. The first two characteristics are incorporated into the model using a result from the previous two chapters: that the population health payoff to the strategy of reimbursement is the net effect of adoption and displacement. More specifically, the model uses the economic payoff to the reimbursement decision, $NEBh^R$: the net population effect of adoption and displacement net the effect of the best alternative strategy. This ensures that the payoff to reimbursement will identify whether it is the population health-maximising strategy and not simply one with a net population health effect greater than zero. This payoff is analogous to the use of economic rent as the payoff to firms in economic models, rather than accounting profit, and is consistent with the objective of maximising population health. (See Sect. 7.6 for a discussion of the net economic benefit.) The third characteristic, strategic behaviour, is incorporated by using a GTM rather than a DTM. The use of a GTM allows the reimbursement problem to be analysed as a high stakes game, where small changes in the decision threshold can result in a significant change in profits for firms and health for the population.

8.3   The High Stakes Game of New Drug Reimbursement

Firms hold patents for their new drugs. Patents are a policy (legislation) intended to correct for the failure of the market to provide an incentive to invest in R&D. Patents achieve this objective by providing market exclusivity; no other firms can produce the patented item unless they are licensed by the patent holder. However, patents also create market power and therefore the patent holding firm is not necessarily a price taker, unlike a firm in a perfectly competitive market. So economic theory suggests we ask: Why would we assume that a firm with market power will offer the new drug at an IPER substantially below the Reimburser's threshold when: (1) it knows that the Reimburser will make the same decision (reimburse for the target group) at a higher price; and (2) no other firm will compete and offer the drug at a lower price?[4]

---

[3] Whether or not above marginal cost pricing is justified by the need to cover the fixed costs of R&D (historic and/or future) is a separate issue addressed in Chaps. 9 and 10. The point here is simply that, once the drug has been developed, it will only be unprofitable to produce it if the price is below marginal cost of production. In the absence of perfect competition there is no pressure from other firms to lower the price if the price is above the marginal cost of production. Therefore, provided that the maximum price is not lowered below the marginal cost of production, it will remain profitable for the Firm to produce the drug at the lower price.

[4] We could also ask why the monopsonist purchaser does not bargain with the producer to identify the price at which the producer will no longer sell. One reason is strategy; bargaining games tend to

Unlike the situation in a perfectly competitive market, where at any point in time there is only one price a profit-maximising firm can charge for a given item (the market price), market power means that firms can (and must) select a price strategically. In this case, "strategically" means the monopolist firm makes reference to the expected response by a monopsonist purchaser in the domestic market to possible offer prices. Given the presence of strategic behaviour, the economic model used to characterise the reimbursement process in this section is game theoretic rather than a DTM. How does a GTM differ from a DTM? And why aren't GTMs used in pharmaco-economics?

8.3.1 Game Theoretic vs. Decision Theoretic Models

Games grow in the spaces where perfect competition does not exist. In perfect competition, the consumers and sellers are price takers and there is no reward for investment in strategic behaviour. In contrast, where the firm and/or the institution have market power, there is a potential for rewards from strategic behaviour. In the case of a new drug, the outcome of the game is the allocation of the economic surplus (value) from clinical innovation between the firm and the institution as agent of consumers. The IPER of the new drug is the mechanism by which this allocation of surplus occurs and a share of this surplus is the possible reward for strategic behaviour. The decision threshold signalled by the institution is a key piece of information (and decision) which, if varied, can change the outcome of the game (the allocation of the innovative surplus) by changing the equilibrium price.

There are two elements common to DTMs and GTMs: (1) decision and chance nodes; and (2) the outcomes of these nodes. However, there is a fundamental difference in the structure and solutions of DTMs compared with GTMs: the latter predict the equilibrium set of actions and strategies, given the interactions between the players each with specific preferences, whereas the former predict which strategy will be preferred by a single decision maker, given his or her preferences. Decision analysis can be characterised as the use of a model to select the optimal action of a single decision maker faced with choices with or without uncertainty

---

have outcomes which result in a share of the surplus being appropriated by each player, unless there is a rule or threat that results in a corner solution (see Watson 2002, pp. 170–203) The second reason is that information on the threshold is in the public domain (or can be inferred from historic decisions) whereas the cost of production is in the private domain and varies across drugs. The third reason is the particular rules of reimbursement processes such as those in Australia. In Australia, the firm is required to provide evidence of the incremental cost and effect, and to demonstrate it is cost-effective (at or below the threshold). If the drug is not cost-effective, the Reimburser could signal that the firm should lower the price until it becomes cost-effective. There is no lever beyond this threshold that can be invoked by the Reimburser. This, as I argue later in this chapter, is what the CEO of Roche is referring to in the quotation at the start of this chapter: "the health economics holds up", that is, if the only criterion for a new drug to be reimbursed is to be cost-effective, then why would it lower the price below this threshold.

(chance nodes). In contrast, game theory can be characterised as being concerned with the equilibrium outcomes of strategic interactions of two or more decision makers, with or without uncertainty. Significantly, the equilibrium outcome of a game is not necessarily the optimal outcome for either or both players. In contrast, the lone decision maker in a DTM is selecting the optimal strategy from a number of strategies in order to maximise (or minimise) expected outcomes. There are no other players influencing choice, therefore, the preferred strategy is always implemented. Hence, the result of a DTM is always the selection of the strategy with the best expected outcome for that decision maker.

This fundamental difference is expressed in the structure of the respective models. Both GTMs and DTMs typically have more than one outcome for each decision (for example, cost and effect). The task of decision analysis is for one decision maker to accommodate multiple outcomes, which might need to be traded against each other (for example, additional costs and additional effect). The additional task of game theoretic analysis is to accommodate multiple objective functions (for example, the firm vs. the consumer).

8.3.2 Examples of Published Pharma-Economic Games

There are very few published GTMs of the drug pricing process in either the pharma-economic or the pharmaco-economic literature. Two examples in recent years analyse aspects of the drug reimbursement process (Wright 2004; Antonanzas et al. 2011). A third game analyses the decision by firms to conduct head-to-head comparative trials of their drugs and the role of incentives in changing the predicted no-trial equilibrium outcomes (Mansley et al. 2007). This game is not discussed further in this book but it provides a powerful example of the relationship between expected profit and strategic choices in the design of clinical trials. It is a rigorous game theoretic approach to analysing the question of "why don't we have more head-to-head clinical trials?"[5]

Wright (2004) presented the process of drug bargaining in Australia as a five-stage game of complete information. Wright was particularly interested in the welfare implications of regulating the price below the Firm's[6] offer price, bargaining when firms can be differentiated in terms of their quality (high for innovative or low for generic); and a single drug having differential impacts in two patient groups. Wright's game identified conditions under which certain firms (high quality firms) could benefit from price regulation. It also identified situations

---

[5] This game about optimal trial design from a strategic perspective is probably the most intuitively accessible of these three games, from the perspective of a pharmaco-economist. The Risk Sharing game is also accessible. Both illustrate the idea of characterising players and their actions.

[6] The Firm is a player in a game and a capital letter is used to signify this particular use of the term. Players have particular characteristics, defined mathematically, and firms with a small "f" do not necessarily have these characteristics.

under which leakage[7] would not reduce a Regulator's surplus. Wright structured his model such that the two initial options for the Firm are: (1) to have its price regulated (below what would otherwise be charged) but subsidised to the consumer; or (2) for the price to be unregulated and unsubsidised. There is a trade-off inherent in the decision to approach the Reimburser; maintain unit price or increase sales. This option does not seem to be relevant to the Australian setting where almost all firms request reimbursement for drugs that are prescribed outside the hospital setting. However, it is possible that Wright is referring to a situation where, for a few drugs, the PBAC will not reimburse the drug at the offer price due to lack of evidence of effect or unacceptable cost-effectiveness. In this case the Firm is effectively choosing to not lower the price it sells the drug at and have the price to consumers subsidised. Instead it is choosing to maintain the higher price and sell to a market where the financial barrier to access for a consumer could be high.[8] Wright does not refer to the presence of a decision threshold nor does the model include a concept of expressing a drug price as an ICER. He refers to prices per course being equivalent across drugs within the same therapeutic group regardless of their "quality".

Wright's model is a reminder that drug price is endogenous not exogenous to the decision process. He also points out that there is an opportunity for firms to use lobbying to extract more of the surplus associated with the reimbursement of the drug, once the firm has agreed to a regulated price. This lobbying for higher prices occurs even though the "high quality firm" in Wright's model is better off by accepting the regulated price in order to gain market share through subsidised drug prices for consumers than by a choosing higher price with no consumer subsidy. Wright concludes that Pharma's "hostility" to regulation and claim that it reduces profit is a strategy to "extract more of the total surplus generated by regulation." (p. 810)

However, a second conclusion is less useful in the context of a reimbursement process that uses economic evaluation, decision thresholds and ICERs. Wright observes that the use of regulation has the objective of improving equity however,

---

[7] Leakage is a term used to describe the practice by prescribers of prescribing to all patients for whom there is a possible therapeutic benefit not just the patients for whom a subsidy has been approved on the grounds that it is cost-effective. The effect of leakage is to increase the budget for that drug beyond the expected expenditure and increase the aICER in actual practice above what was expected due to decreasing marginal benefits and increasing marginal costs.

[8] It's complicated. If we assume that all drugs with acceptable cost-effectiveness are reimbursed at the offer price, then the benefits of a firm choosing not to have a drug reimbursed and instead sell it unsubsidised to consumers would appear limited, particularly if the new drug is very high cost. Furthermore, to sell a drug that is not subsidised when it is demonstrated to not be "value for money" would appear to be a strategy with little value. However, what is acceptable to a firm might not be acceptable to the regulator. Firms and regulators would dispute whether there are any new drugs that are not reimbursed that have acceptable evidence to support their evidence of incremental cost and effect, and have an acceptable ICER. Hence it is difficult if not impossible to count the number of drugs that meet these criteria of evidence quality and ICER acceptability and are not listed (subsidised) because the firm is unwilling to sell at that cost-effective price.

it also has efficiency implications. He argues that because regulation results in a single price across drugs with varying quality but in the same therapeutic group, these efficiency implications are not desirable.

In fact, groups of drugs with a single price per course and in the same drug class are typically all generics (or all on patent). If a drug is of higher quality (which is assumed to mean more effective than a comparator) and is on patent, then it will have a higher price per course if it prices at an ICER above zero.[9] Furthermore, improving equity (in access by consumers through a co-payment scheme) is a different decision from the maximum price an institution should pay for the incremental health effects of a new drug. Wright's paper provides some insights but does not assist in the choice of a single threshold for new drugs based on their incremental cost and effect.

For their research on the conditions under which a regulator and a firm would both have an incentive for a risk sharing agreement[10] (RSA) for a new drug of uncertain benefit, Antonanzas et al. (2011) characterised two possible contracts between Firms and Regulators: RSAs and non-RSAs. In their GTM of complete information, the stylised RSAs required Regulators to pay Firms only if a patient is cured whereas non-RSAs require payment to the Firm per patient treated, regardless of the observable response by patients. The paper established the conditions under which the preferences of the Firm and the Regulators would be aligned and a contract (either RSA or non-RSA) would be mutually preferable. They found that if drugs have a relatively low cost impact, health funders will prefer not to risk share, and with high cost impact drugs and low costs of monitoring they would prefer an RSA.

8.3.3   Why Aren't Games Used in Pharmaco-Economic Models?

The pharmaco-economic literature has a rich tradition of DTMs but not GTMs. A possible explanation is that pharmaco-economics occupies the only space in the reimbursement process within which there is no strategic behaviour. This space is the (non-strategic) behaviour of the new molecule given patient characteristics, dose and duration of therapy. All other aspects of the new drug involve strategic behaviour, including the generation of evidence from clinical trials, the construction of pharmaco-economic models to maximise the possible additional benefit and minimise the additional cost; the offer price selected by the firms, and the recruitment of key clinicians for post-marketing studies.

---

[9] A cursory review of the PBS schedule in a class with both generics and on-patent drugs indicates that the price per course is not identical.

[10] The highest profile RSA is that between the UK regulators and the firms that owned the patent for a range of drugs for Multiple Sclerosis (Boggild et al. 2009).

The dominance of DTMs in HTA/CEA can be characterised as a consequence of pharmaco-economic research addressing the market's failure to summarise the complex information about the health and cost consequences of adopting a new drug at a given drug offer price. DTMs can accommodate and analyse uncertainty in parameters and the impact of uncertainty on optimal decision-making. Therefore, DTMs are the model of choice to solve for the IPER of a new drug, which can then be used in the reimbursement process. However, information about the IPER of a new drug at a given price is not the only information the market fails to provide. DTMs cannot correct for the failure of the market to reveal an IPER generated by the firm that reflects competition in the market for health inputs. This market failure is a consequence of the market power of the seller that arises from patents and the market power of a monopsonist purchaser. For an economic model to be used to analyse this aspect of the real world, it needs to incorporate strategic behaviour.

In summary, molecules do not act strategically, therefore it is appropriate to use DTMs to analyse the consequences (costs and effects) of new drug adoption. They can be used to estimate the IPER of a new drug at a given price and accommodate the associated uncertainty. However, DTMs cannot be used to analyse situations in which people, firms and institutions act strategically when they buy, sell, prescribe and consume these molecules. Therefore DTMs can be used to inform, but not analyse, the decision to reimburse the drug. The Game described in the following section illustrates how strategic behaviour by players with market power can be accommodated in an economic model.

8.4   The New Drug Reimbursement Game

The drug reimbursement game presented in this chapter is far less ambitious than the three published games described above; its aim is to demonstrate new drug price as an equilibrium outcome of reimbursement rather than an exogenous choice by the Firm. It was developed using Grüne-Yanoff and Schweinzer's (GY-S) Architecture of Game Theory (Grüne-Yanoff and Schweinzer 2008). This architecture characterises game theory as having three components: World, the Model and Theory Proper.

"World" characterises the economic situation which, in an applied economic model, is the justification for the analysis. "Model" comprises a Narrative and a Game Structure. The Narrative is the story that sets out the players, the ordering of events and the justifications for their payoffs. It also clarifies the opportunities for the players to act strategically. The Game Structure is analogous to the decision tree in a DTM. (For example compare the decision tree presented in Fig. 8.1 with the extensive form game presented in Fig. 8.2 in Sect. 8.6.2.1) The Game Structure also includes the formal expression of all the payoffs, conditions, assumptions and parameters. Theory Proper is the theoretical foundation of the problem. Solution Concepts can be thought of as theory expressed as a rule that is used to predict how a player or game will be played. This is most commonly an equilibrium concept, the most well-known of which is the Nash Equilibrium. (See Watson 2002)

The Game's Narrative, which precedes the Game Structure in a formal expression of the overall problem, is a detailed qualitative description of the Game. The Narrative's role in the GTM can be thought of as analogous to the body of empirical evidence and associated narratives that support the pharmaco-economic model, as distinct from the technical assumptions in the model.

Grüne-Yanoff and Schweinzer describe a given economic situation as having multiple interpretations and hence solutions.[11] The authors describe the role of the Narrative in supporting a game's solution by directing which of the many possible solution concepts should be applied, hence selecting a concept of rationality from the many possible rather than defining a unique rationality.

Accordingly, the Game presented in this chapter is designed to have sufficient detail in the Narrative to support the Solution Concepts used in the Game, but other concepts.

8.5 World (The Economic Problem)

The Reimburser is about to apply β_c as the threshold IPER where:

$$\beta_c = \left(\frac{1}{n} - \frac{1}{m} + \frac{1}{d}\right)^{-1}.$$

The use of a health shadow price that accommodates the characteristics of the health care sector appeals to the Reimburser. She recognises that allocative inefficiency is a significant feature of health care budgets throughout the OECD (Garber and Skinner 2008). The Reimburser also recognises that there is no Institution analogous to reimbursing institutions that make systematic improvements to allocative efficiency by reallocating funds across existing programmes and technologies (Culyer et al. 2007; Elshaug et al. 2007; Pearson and Littlejohns 2007). She also recognises that displacement could be suboptimal $(d < m)$ and that suboptimality of displacement is not a parameter she can control.

Then the Reimburser thinks about this threshold IPER from the perspective of the Firm. At \$5,042 per QALY, β_c is significantly lower than the threshold of \$75,000 per QALY she used historically. She wonders whether the clinicians are

---

[11] This particular idea of multiple solutions is distinct from the idea of a non-unique solution to a given problem. The authors describe this idea as each solution concept capturing a specific notion of rationality and that game theory tools offer to "model specific situations at varying degrees and kinds of rationality". Narratives have a role in supporting the particular rationality being used to solve a given game. Hence, the multiple solutions are a consequence of multiple rationalities, whereas non-unique solutions refer to the consequences of a single rationality.

correct: will this lower maximum price mean that drugs that would otherwise have been reimbursed at prices above \$5,042 per QALY will no longer be reimbursed? The Reimburser considers the idea of the opportunity cost of these additional high cost drugs. She wonders: if fewer new drugs are available as a consequence, will the population necessarily be worse off than it would have been under the existing maximum IPER of \$75,000 per QALY?

The Reimburser asks her Health Economic Adviser how the Institution should respond to the following threat:

- If the threshold is reduced from \$75,000 to $\beta_c = \$5,024$ per QALY, less than 15 % of the new drugs that would otherwise be approved will be made available to patients. The population will be worse off at the lower threshold IPER.

8.6   Model

The model comprises the Narrative and the Game Structure.

8.6.1   Narrative

The Narrative comprises the Firm's decision, the Institution's decision and the rules of new drug reimbursement.

8.6.1.1   The Firm's Decision

A pharmaceutical firm (the Firm) completes the R&D cycle for a hypothetical new drug for rheumatoid arthritis called Araamax and now two regulatory hurdles need to be cleared. The first hurdle is regulatory approval for clinicians to prescribe Araamax for certain groups of patients. The evidence required for this hurdle is that of the comparative clinical effectiveness of the drug. Specifically, it needs to be demonstrated in a clinical trial that the new drug is no worse than the best existing drug for that condition. We assume that the patent holders have demonstrated that Araamax has superiority (an additional health gain for target patients) against the existing drug (Rathmab) in an appropriate clinical trial; it is clinically innovative. Furthermore, the group of patients for whom Araamax represents a clinical benefit (the target patients) all have the same incremental benefit compared with the best existing therapy and no patients outside this group experience a benefit from this drug.

The second hurdle is approval for government reimbursement of the costs of Araamax for a patient for whom it is prescribed. This approval is for reimbursing the entire cost of Araamax for all patients for whom prescribing is approved (the target group). The evidence required to clear the reimbursement hurdle is that of the price of the new drug expressed as the additional financial cost to the health sector per additional unit of health effect, or in PEA terminology, the IPER. The estimate of this IPER (the evidence) is produced by the Firm and is public information in the context of the Game; it is known to both the Institution and the Firm.

Araamax is patented and, as a monopolist, the Firm needs to select rather than accept the price at which it offers the new drug to the reimbursement authority. We assume it selects the price so as to maximise economic profit.

There are two factors that the Firm needs to take into consideration when selecting an offer price: the marginal cost of production of the drug (which defines the minimum price at which the Firm will be willing to produce the drug) and the Institution's signal of the threshold IPER; the maximum price the Institution is willing to pay for a new health effect. Each of these are discussed in detail in the following sections.

The Marginal Cost of Production of Araamax

Tables 8.1 to 8.6 set out a "worked example" of the relationships between clinical innovation, price, costs of manufacturing and economic rents. (Corresponding numbers are presented in the text in italics, bracketed and referenced to the tables. These numbers are not used in the model, which is solved algebraically. These numbers are simply illustrative of cost concepts.)

In this example, incremental measures are compared with their own next best alternative therapy (Rathmab to placebo; and Araamax to Rathmab) and Araamax is also compared to placebo. Three firm related variables are illustrated.

- The IPER is the conventional ICER for the drugs, but is referred to as an IPER to capture the endogeneity of price.
- The incremental manufacturing cost-effectiveness ratio (IMER) is a ratio of the additional costs of manufacturing the new drug to the additional QALYs of the new drug compared with the next best alternative. A new drug could have clinical innovation, but the costs of producing the new drug are the same as the cost of producing the older drug and hence the IMER could be zero.
- The incremental economic profit effectiveness ratio IπER is the incremental economic rent derived by the Firm per incremental QALY, at a given IPER and IMER.

In this case we assume that Rathmab, which will be entirely replaced by Araamax, is off-patent and priced at the marginal cost of production, which is constant ($250 (a))—where (a) references the corresponding cell in Table 8.4. As is conventional in economics, the marginal cost of production includes a cost that

Table 8.1 QALYs per course per patient

Comparison	Incremental QALYs per patient
Rathmab vs. placebo	0.05
Araamax vs. Rathmab	0.07
Araamax vs. placebo	0.12[a]

[a]The clinical innovation of Araamax compared to placebo (0.12) contains 0.05 QALYs that are innovation from Rathmab compared to placebo.

Table 8.2 IPER (incremental price per incremental QALY) per course

Comparison	IPER ($)
Rathmab vs. placebo	5,000
Araamax vs. Rathmab	75,000
Araamax vs. Placebo	45,833[a]

[a]The IPER of each drug weighted by each drug's clinical innovation relative to own best alternative therapy.

Table 8.3 Expenditure per course

Comparison	Cost of a course ($)[a]
Additional cost of a course of Rathmab vs. placebo = cost of a course of Rathmab	250
Additional cost of a course of Araamax compared to Rathmab	5,250
Additional cost of a course of Rathmab vs. placebo = cost of a course of Araamax	5,500

[a]The total cost of a course of drugs is derived from the product of the number of QALYs per course for one patient (Table 8.1) and the cost per QALY for each drug (Table 8.2). The drugs are the only financial cost of care.

Table 8.4 Cost of manufacture per course

Cost of a course ($)	
Rathmab	250(a)[a]
Araamax	250(a)[b]

[a]The cost of manufacturing a course of Rathmab is the same as the price because it is a generic; it is priced at its marginal cost of production, which includes normal profit.
[b]The cost of manufacturing a course of Araamax and Rathmab are the same.(a) corresponds to a reference in the text above these tables.

Table 8.5 Per course summary measures

Per course summary measures	Rathmab	Araamax
QALY	0.05	0.12
Price	250	5,500
Cost of manufacture	250	250
Economic rent	0	5,250

The key indicators for the drugs are summarised on a per course basis where the comparator is placebo. For example, the health gain per course of Rathmab is simply the health gains compared to placebo for a patient.

Table 8.6 Per incremental QALY summary measures

Per incremental QALY measures	Description	Rathmab vs. placebo	Araamax vs. Rathmab
IPER	Incremental price per incremental QALY	5,000[a]	75,000 (b)
IMER	Incremental cost of manufacture per incremental QALY	5,000[b]	0 (b)
IπER[c]	Incremental economic rent per incremental QALY = IPER—IMER in this case	0	75,000 (b)

[a]*Rathmab vs. placebo*: The IPER for Rathmab is the same as the IMER because the drug is off-patent

[b]*Araamax vs. Rathmab*: The IMER captures the additional costs of manufacturing the additional QALYs for Araamax vs. Rathmab. In this case there is no additional cost of manufacturing Araamax therefore the IMER is 0

[c]The IπER is the incremental economic rent per incremental QALY. It is 0 for the off-patent drug and the same as the IPER for Araamax.(*b*) refers to the text in this section

represents normal profits (or the opportunity cost of resources owned by the firm).[12] Furthermore, we assume that the marginal cost of producing Araamax is constant across quantity and the same as the marginal cost of producing a course of Rathmab (*$250 (a)* Table 8.4). Finally, we assume that the only cost consequence to the health budget of financing Araamax is its additional cost compared with Rathmab; there are no other resource implications. Therefore, Araamax's IPER relative to Rathmab represents the Firm's economic rent on each unit of effect purchased by the Institution. (*$75,000 (b)* Table 8.6)

Maximum Acceptable Price

The second factor the Firm needs to consider is the Institution's maximum acceptable IPER for the health gains from the new drug. Unlike conventional market situations, the Firm does not need to consider the price elasticity of demand for the new drug between the maximum acceptable price and the marginal cost of production. This situation exists because, if the Institution adopts the drug, the full cost of the drug is reimbursed for all target patients and no other patients. Therefore the quantity of the drug that will be purchased will be the same, regardless of the price at which it was adopted, provided that price is less than or equal to the Institution's maximum acceptable price. This situation, infinite price elasticity of demand below the maximum acceptable price and perfect price elasticity above this price, leads to the potential quantity of sales (measured in health effects) as either fixed at the expected incremental health effect for the target patient group $\overline{\Delta E^p}$ or zero.

---

[12] When economists refer to economic profit they are referring to profit that is over and above the opportunity cost of a firm's capital, hence the Economics 101 result of the perfectly competitive market: "All firms earn zero profits in the long run competitive equilibrium." For an explanation without the maths, see Landsburg (1988) pp. 191–193.

8.6.1.2   The Institution's Decision

Reimbursement in a fixed budget involves both adoption and displacement. The adoption of a new clinically innovative drug has the result of increasing the health of the target patients compared with the therapy they would otherwise have received. However, adopting the new drug involves an additional financial cost to the health care system compared with usual therapy. The Institution's budget is fixed, therefore this additional financial cost of the new drug must be financed by displacing existing health services. Displacing these services leads to a loss in health effects for the population.

In order to finance the additional costs of a new drug, other agents in the health system will displace unpatented services. Displacement can be suboptimal; the least cost-effective in contraction of current programmes are not necessarily the ones that are displaced; this is outside the control of the reimbursing Institution. The Institution wants to avoid a situation where the gains from the new drug are considered in isolation from the health effects lost by displacing services. Therefore the Institution defines the net health effect of reimbursement as the net health effect for the population: the increase in the health of the target patients who are prescribed the new drug, less the loss in health for patients whose services are displaced to finance the new drug:

$$\Delta E^R = \overline{\Delta E^p} - \Delta E^D.$$

There are constraints around the displacement process. The only health services that can be displaced are those that are unpatented. These services, which consist mainly of labour inputs, include respite care and rehabilitation. These programmes are infinitely divisible; the budget for a given programme can be reduced or increased by the smallest increment. Furthermore, if the budget is reduced, both the inputs, for example labour, and the output (effect measured in QALYs) are also reduced. This means the outcome of displacement is continuous; any amount can be displaced and any change in this amount will change the health effects for this group of patients. The aICER of a given programme is assumed to be constant, regardless of programme size, but varies across programmes. We assume the estimate of the aICER of these programmes is certain—an assumption that is relaxed in the Conclusion to this book. Furthermore, the services that are displaced are not necessarily the least cost-effective of existing services. Displacement is exogenous (outside the control of the reimbursing Institution) and possibly suboptimal; it could be any mix of the least and most cost-effective existing unpatented services.[13]

---

[13] The somewhat stochastic process of displacing existing service to finance new drugs tends to be a less directed largely politically determined process than reimbursement. It might be spread over many smaller programs and described as "budget cut-backs". There are no Institutions analogous to the reimbursement Institutions that systematically determine whether a given service or technology should be disinvested (planned contraction of programs), although there is an

Other pharmaceuticals cannot be displaced to finance the additional costs of new drugs because the decision to reimburse them protects them by law from displacement; however, if a new more effective drug is developed and reimbursed for the target patients then the existing drug will be completely replaced. The loss in health gains due to replacement of the previous drug is incorporated in the clinical payoff for the new drug because the clinical innovation of the new drug is compared with the best available therapy for these patients.

The Institution is also concerned about the foregone benefit of alternative ways of accessing and allocating health budget funds. The Institution is aware that the budget is currently allocatively inefficient and that in such a situation: (1) the best alternative strategy to reimbursement could be reallocation across programmes; and (2) the foregone benefit of funds allocated to new drug purchases could be significant. An amount of funds can be reallocated from Programme M, the least cost-effective (in contraction) of currently financed programmes, to Programme N, the most cost-effective (in expansion). The foregone benefits of this alternative strategy can be internalised in the reimbursement decision as a forgone benefit in the payoff to reimbursement. Hence the Institution chooses an economic net benefit (the net health gains from reimbursement less the health gains from optimal reallocation) as the payoff to reimbursement. This choice is analogous to economists' preference for using economic rent rather than accounting profit as a firm's payoff. Accounting profit is revenue less costs of manufacturing, whereas economic rent is revenue less the cost of manufacturing and normal profit. A firm can have an accounting profit but an economic loss if the profit from the best alternative strategy is more than that from the strategy of manufacturing drugs. A profit-maximising firm will not manufacture if it expects an economic loss, even if it has an accounting profit, because it would be better off taking the more profitable alternative strategy.

If the Institution is indifferent between reimbursement and doing nothing, we assume it is required to reimburse the new drug. This requirement is a consequence of legislation.

8.6.1.3 The Rules of Reimbursement and Other Parts to the Story

1. The narrative describing the Firm's and Institution's decisions contains a number of references to the Institution's rules.
2. The Game starts when the Firm offers the new drug at a price expressed as an IPER; the Institution never approaches the Firm with an offer price.
3. The reimbursement process comprises adoption (of the new drug) and displacement (of existing non-patented services).

---

increasing interest in establishing such a process (Pearson and Littlejohns 2007). It is proposed such processes would be driven by the evidence of a program or technology's lack of effect (e.g. some surgical procedures).

4. Only non-patented services and programmes can be displaced by the Institution to finance the additional cost of the new patented drug. Patented inputs are protected by the existing reimbursement processes.
5. Displacement is exogenous to the reimbursing Institution and not necessarily optimal.
6. The choice to adopt or not adopt the new drug has a discrete outcome, 0 or $\overline{\Delta E^p}$ (not adopt means no impact, and adopt means an increase in health), whereas both the action and outcome of displacement are continuous (the programme can be contracted or expanded by any amount).
7. If the Institution is indifferent between reimbursement and rejection, it must reimburse.
8. The Institution wants to avoid a situation where the health gains from the new drug are considered in isolation from the health effects lost by other patients as a consequence of displacement.
9. The Institution is aware that current allocation is inefficient and that the processes for reallocation are not institutionalised in the same way that drug reimbursement is.
10. There is *no relationship* between the new drug's price and future innovation. (This assumption is relaxed in the following two chapters.)

8.6.1.4   The Threat

• If the threshold is reduced to β_c, less than 15 % of the new drugs that would otherwise be approved will be made available to patients. The population's health will be worse as a result.

8.6.2   Game Structure

8.6.2.1   Extensive Form Representation of the Game

The extensive form representation of the game is presented in Fig. 8.2.

8.6.2.2   Players, Actions and Payoffs

The players are the pharmaceutical firm (Firm, F) and the reimbursing institution (Institution, I), the health care budget holder. The Game is initiated when the Firm brings a new pharmaceutical to the Institution.

The Firm's action is to choose a price, $f \in (0, \infty)$. (In Fig. 8.2 the arc representing the Firm's choice indicates that there is a set of possible prices from which it selects one.) The Institution's action is $a_i \in (R, N)$, where: R is reimburse (adopt and displace) and N is do nothing.

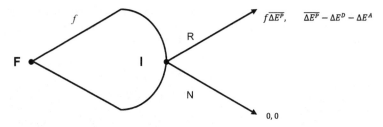

Fig. 8.2 The new drug reimbursement game

If the Institution chooses to reimburse the new drug the payoffs are:

- (*To the Firm*) $f\overline{\Delta E^P}$, the economic rent to the Firm,

  - where f is the IPER and $\overline{\Delta E^P}$ is the clinical innovation of the new drug for all target patients compared with best available care; and

- (*To the Institution*) $\text{NEBh}^R = \Delta E^R - \Delta E^A = \overline{\Delta E^P} - \Delta E^D - \Delta E^A$, the net economic benefit (health) to the population

  - Where $\overline{\Delta E^P} - \Delta E^D$ is the net effect of displacement and adoption (the net effect on population health); and
  - ΔE^A is the foregone benefit of improved allocative efficiency (the best alternative strategy given that the budget is allocatively inefficient).

If the Institution chooses to do nothing there is no payoff to either the Firm or the Institution. The payoffs to both the Firm and the Institution are economic payoffs; therefore, we can conclude that, if these payoffs are positive, there is no better action available to the players.

8.6.2.3 Parameters and Variables

- ΔE^P is the health effect of the new drug.

  - The drug can only be adopted for all, not some, of the eligible patients.
  - $\overline{\Delta E^P}$ is the total additional health effect for all patients eligible for the new drug.
  - ΔE^P can take two values: $\overline{\Delta E^P}$ (if the drug is adopted); and 0 (if the drug is rejected).

- ΔE^D is the health effect displaced in order to finance the additional cost of the new drug.
- ΔE^A is the net gain in population health from reallocation of resources from Programme M to Programme N.
- f is the IPER of the new drug.

The parameters and variables that describe the payoffs of the actions available to the Institution can be specified in terms of the total cost and unit cost of achieving them.

- $$\overline{\Delta E^P} = \frac{\Delta C^P}{f}$$

  – Is the additional health effect for target patients if the drug is adopted,
  – Where ΔC^P is the additional financial cost to the health care budget of financing the additional effects from the new drug: $\overline{\Delta E^P}$ at an IPER of f.

- $$\Delta E^D = \frac{\Delta C^P}{d}$$

  – Is the health effect displaced because services are displaced to finance ΔC^P, where d is the aICER of the services displaced to finance the new drug.

- $\Delta E^A = \Delta E^N - \Delta E^M$ is the net gain in population health effects from reallocation of resources, ΔC^P from Programme M to Programme N.

  – where n and m are the aICERs of Programmes N and M in expansion and contraction, respectively.

- $$\Delta E^N = \frac{\Delta C^P}{n}$$

  – where ΔE^N is the additional health effect available when the variable cost budget for Programme N is expanded by an amount ΔC^P.

- $$\Delta E^M = \frac{\Delta C^P}{m}$$

  – where ΔE^M is the health effect lost when Programme M's budget is contracted by amount ΔC^P.

- $\Delta E^R = \overline{\Delta E^P} - \Delta E^D$ is the net gain to the population from Strategy R (adoption and displacement).

Finally, the economic rent to the Firm at price f is determined by the Firm's production function. The Firm's additional cost of production for the additional health gains compared with the existing drug (the IMER) is zero. This is the situation because: (1) the marginal cost of production of the new drug is the same as for the off-patent drug that the new drug will replace; and (2) the existing drug is priced at its marginal cost of production. The marginal cost of production includes the forgone benefit of the Firm's best alternative production options. Therefore, any payment the Firm receives for the additional health gains of the new drug compared to usual care represent economic rent. This situation is illustrated in Fig. 8.2 where the generic drug is priced at the marginal cost of production and has a financial profit that is also a normal profit.

- $\pi = f\overline{\Delta E^p}$ is the economic rent available to the Firm.

8.6.2.4 Conditions

- $\overline{\Delta E^p} > 0$. The drug brought to the Institution is clinically innovative, that is, it has a clinical advantage compared with the best available existing therapy for the target group of patients. The health gain is fixed (discrete) for the identified group of target patients, and is known with certainty.
- $d > 0$. The aICER of the services displaced to finance the additional financial costs of the new drug is greater than zero.
- $\Delta E^D > 0$. It follows from $d > 0$ that displacing services to finance the additional costs of the new drug will lead to a loss in health effects for patients who would otherwise have received these services.
- ΔE^D is continuous. The funding to the displaced services can be reduced or increased by the smallest increment. If the funding is changed, the effect will change in the same direction.
- $f \geq 0$. The price per additional effect of the new drug compared to the best available therapy is greater than or equal to zero.
- $\Delta C^P \geq 0$. The additional financial cost to the health budget of the new drug is greater than or equal to zero. This condition is a consequence of the previous assumptions: $\overline{\Delta E^p}$, $f \geq 0$.
- $\Delta E^A > 0$. The health care budget is currently allocatively inefficient, therefore optimal reallocation results in a net gain in health effects.
- $m > n > 0$. There is allocative inefficiency.

8.7 Theory Proper

This game draws on economic theory relating to the pricing decisions made by the profit-maximising monopolistic Firm that takes into account both its own and the Institution's payoff. We recognise that the only decision that a rational Institution can make is to select an appropriate payoff (the net economic benefit), which it then needs to apply in the reimbursement decision. The Solution Concept used to solve the game is backward induction.[14]

8.8 Solution

Using backward induction, assuming all terminal nodes can be reached, we solve the game starting from the outcomes of the last stages.

8.8.1 Stage 2: The Institution's Decision

What decision rules will the Institution use to provide a response to any possible IPER offered by the Firm?

- If $\overline{\Delta E^P} - \Delta E^D - \Delta E^A < 0$, the Institution will choose the action "do Nothing" (N).
- If $\overline{\Delta E^P} - \Delta E^D - \Delta E^A \geq 0$, the Institution will choose "Reimburse" (R).

Hence, the critical price above which the Institution will reject, and at or below which it will reimburse, is calculated as follows.

First, we obtain an expression for the population health effects from reallocation:

$$\Delta E^A = \Delta E^N - \Delta E^M,$$

where

$$\Delta E^N = \frac{\Delta C^P}{n} \text{ and } \Delta E^M = \frac{\Delta C^P}{m}$$

$$\therefore \Delta E^A = \Delta C^P \left(\frac{1}{n} - \frac{1}{m} \right) \tag{8.1}$$

is the gain in health to the population from the strategy of reallocation.

The point of indifference between Strategy R and Strategy N (the decision threshold) occurs when:

---

[14] Watson (2002) defines the solution concept of backward induction as analysing a game by starting at the end of the game and working back and identifying and "striking out" any action that is dominated and leaving the terminal nodes that can be reached.

$$\left(\overline{\Delta E^P} - \Delta E^D\right) - \Delta E^A = 0.$$

Substituting this in Eq. (8.1)

$$\therefore \overline{\Delta E^P} - \Delta E^D - \Delta C^P \left(\frac{1}{n} - \frac{1}{m}\right) = 0,$$

where

$$\overline{\Delta E^P} = \frac{\Delta C^P}{f}$$

and

$$\Delta E^D = \frac{\Delta C^P}{d}$$

$$\Rightarrow \frac{\Delta C^P}{f} - \frac{\Delta C^P}{d} - \Delta C^P \left(\frac{1}{n} - \frac{1}{m}\right) = 0,$$

and as $\Delta C > 0$

$$\Rightarrow \frac{1}{f} - \frac{1}{d} - \left(\frac{1}{n} - \frac{1}{m}\right) = 0$$

$$\Rightarrow \frac{1}{f} = \frac{1}{d} + \left(\frac{1}{n} - \frac{1}{m}\right)$$

$$\therefore f = \left(\frac{1}{d} + \left(\frac{1}{n} - \frac{1}{m}\right)\right)^{-1}.$$

So the Institution's decision rule is:

- Reimburse if:

$$f \leq \left(\frac{1}{d} + \left(\frac{1}{n} - \frac{1}{m}\right)\right)^{-1}.$$

- Do Nothing (Reject) if:

$$f > \left(\frac{1}{d} + \left(\frac{1}{n} - \frac{1}{m}\right)\right)^{-1}.$$

This decision rule is consistent with the Institution choosing to reimburse only if the net economic benefit (health or monetary) is greater than or equal to zero, and hence consistent with the objective of maximising the population's health. If the Institution could instead reallocate an amount from Programme M to Programme N and have a greater impact on the population's health compared with reimbursing the new drug, it would reject the drug.

8.8.2 Stage 1: The Firm's Decision

The Firm has a particular profit function as a consequence of the nature of the reimbursement decision. If the Firm prices above the decision threshold, it will not sell any of the drug.[15] If it lowers the price only as far as the decision threshold it will sell the maximum possible quantity. If it lowers its price further, it will not increase the quantity sold, only reduce the IPER and hence reduce the revenue. Therefore, the profit-maximising Firm chooses the corner solution,[16] which in this case is:

$$f = \left(\frac{1}{d} + \left(\frac{1}{n} - \frac{1}{m} \right) \right)^{-1}.$$

8.8.3 Equilibrium Price and Payoff

Here are the equilibrium results of the Game.

- The equilibrium price is:

$$f^* = \left(\frac{1}{d} + \left(\frac{1}{n} - \frac{1}{m} \right) \right)^{-1}. \tag{8.2}$$

---

[15] This Game assumes that the Firm chooses not to lobby for the price to be above the economic threshold, once it has been declared. There are some situations where the Firm can offer a price above the threshold price and then provide a case for this price, for example the high cost of R&D needs to be financed (Chap. 9), that new drugs need a premium over the standard maximum price because Firms invest in future innovative drugs (Chap. 10), or that new drugs have additional qualities beyond health [Pekarsky (2012, Appendix 10)].

[16] In Consumer Theory, an example of the corner solution is when the utility maximising solution occurs when the entire income is allocated to one good rather than across two goods. In this situation—the drug reimbursement game—it is describing an outcome in a case where there is no negotiation to lower the price when an offer price is at the threshold, even if this price could be tolerated by the Firm (it still makes an economic rent). There is no negotiation because the necessary and sufficient condition of this game—the price being at or below the threshold—is met at the IPER = threshold. It is a situation where the outcome is "extreme", given the threshold selected by the Institution.

The equilibrium price is the IPER of the new drug at which the Institution is indifferent between the actions Reimbursement and do Nothing doing and the Firm's economic rent is maximised.

- The net economic payoff to the Firm:

$$\pi = f^* \overline{\Delta E^p} = \overline{\Delta E^p} \left(\frac{1}{d} + \left(\frac{1}{n} - \frac{1}{m} \right) \right)^{-1}.$$

This is the economic profit to the Firm from above marginal cost pricing of every unit of the new drug.

- The net health benefit of reimbursement (population):

$$\Delta E^R = \overline{\Delta E^p} - \Delta E^D$$

$$= \Delta C^P \left(\frac{1}{f^*} - \frac{1}{d} \right)$$

$$= \Delta C^P \left(\left(\frac{1}{d} + \left(\frac{1}{n} - \frac{1}{m} \right) \right) - \frac{1}{d} \right)$$

$$= \Delta C^P \left(\frac{1}{n} - \frac{1}{m} \right).$$

Now: $m > n$ therefore $\Delta E^R > 0$.

This gives a net increase in the health of the population as a consequence of reimbursement. The gain to target patients due to clinical innovation less the health effects displaced to finance the new drug is greater than zero.

- The economic payoff to the Institution at equilibrium:
  The net economic benefit (health) is:

$$\text{NEBh}^R = \overline{\Delta E^p} - \Delta E^D - \Delta E^A,$$

where

$$\overline{\Delta E^p} = \frac{\Delta C^P}{f^*}, \quad \Delta E^D = \frac{\Delta C^P}{d},$$

and
therefore:

$$\Delta E^A = \Delta C^P \left(\frac{1}{n} - \frac{1}{m} \right)$$

$$\text{NEBh}^R = \frac{\Delta C^P}{f^*} - \frac{\Delta C^P}{d} - \Delta C^P \left(\frac{1}{n} - \frac{1}{m} \right)$$

$$= \Delta C^P \left(\frac{1}{f^*} - \frac{1}{d} - \left(\frac{1}{n} - \frac{1}{m} \right) \right),$$

and from Eq. (8.2)

$$f^* = \left(\frac{1}{d} + \left(\frac{1}{n} - \frac{1}{m} \right) \right)^{-1}$$

$$\therefore \frac{1}{f^*} - \frac{1}{d} - \left(\frac{1}{n} - \frac{1}{m} \right) = 0,$$

if both sides are multiplied by ΔC^P then

$$\overline{\Delta E^P} - \Delta E^D - \Delta E^A = 0.$$

That is, the economic payoff to the Institution is zero at the equilibrium price. This is the corner solution. The entire economic value of the clinical surplus of the new drug is appropriated by the Firm. The increase in the health of the target patients is no greater than that which could have been achieved for other patients through reallocation, and hence the net economic benefit (health) of reimbursement at equilibrium is zero.

8.9   Discussion and Conclusion

At the equilibrium price, the Firm is maximising its economic profit by responding to:

- The public information about the Institution's maximum acceptable IPER; and
- The Institution's lack of bargaining power to negotiate a price below this maximum (despite legislation that allows it to regulate the price to one at or below the decision threshold).

Regardless of the Institution's choice of threshold IPER, if it is above the marginal cost of production and there is no other constraint operating on the Firm, the Firm is predicted to price at the threshold IPER. The equilibrium price is endogenous, not exogenous, to the reimbursement process.

8.9.1   The Reimburser's Questions

The Reimburser revisits her questions.

- Will this lower threshold IPER mean that drugs that would otherwise have been reimbursed at prices above $5,042 will no longer be reimbursed?

The GTM predicts that reducing the maximum acceptable IPER will *not necessarily* result in drugs that would otherwise have been priced at the previous maximum acceptable IPER becoming unavailable to the population. The critical metric for the Firm's decision to produce and supply the new drug is whether the

IπER on the additional units of health effects is greater than or equal to zero,(not whether the IPER has increased or decreased relative to previous years). While the revenue to firms will be lower under this lower threshold IPER (assuming the target group of patients and hence total units sold remains constant), firms have market power and can price above their marginal cost of production. Therefore some firms will still be able to produce and supply their drug at the lower threshold IPER with an economic profit. If firms did not have market power (as in the case of the producers of Rathmab), lowering the price per course of the new drug would result in an economic loss (and possibly also an accounting loss) for the firm on each unit sold and the firm would no longer produce that drug. However, patent holders of new drugs have market power, which means that they could have economic rent and hence the capacity to lower their price and remain profitable.

A second issue is that even if the threshold IPER were zero, some firms would still produce and make an economic profit. If the example in Table 8.4 were changed such that the cost of manufacturing a course of Araamax were $100 instead of $250 (including normal profit), then the manufacturer of Araamax would have an economic profit at an IPER of zero. The economic profit would be $150 per course. This occurs because at an IPER of 0 for Araamax (Araamax compared with Rathmab) the price per course of Araamax would be the same as the price per course of Rathmab ($250); the incremental health benefits are obtained at no additional cost to the Institution. However, the cost of manufacturing a course of Araamax is lower (at $100) due to manufacturing innovation. (See Sect. 4.3.2). Hence, the economic rent on a course of Araamax is $150 ($250 − $100). This shows that a firm can have economic rent even if the IPER is zero.

There is a second situation where Araamax can have an economic rent above zero when the IPER is 0. In the case explored in this game, the drug that is being substituted, Rathmab, has an economic rent of zero because it is off patent. However, if Rathmab were still on patent, then economic rent could be payable on the incremental QALYs for Rathmab vs. placebo. In this case, it is possible that the economic rent on the production of Araamax could be even higher than the economic rent from the additional QALYs for Araamax, even if the IMER for Araamax is zero or less than zero. (See Table 8.6) If the IPER for Rathmab were $7,000 then the firm producing Araamax would appropriate this economic rent. It could therefore tolerate an economic loss up to $2,000 per incremental QALY for Araamax vs. Rathmab. Critically, this economic rent would continue to be paid regardless of the patent expiry of Rathmab. That is, the firm producing Araamax is able to appropriate the economic rent from Rathmab long after the patent on Rathmab would have expired, provided it can be priced relative to Rathmab before that patent expires, and the regulator does not attempt to change the price after Rathmab goes off patent. [This issue is discussed in more detail and with reference to the statins market in Pekarsky (2012, Appendix 6).]

- Will this result make the population worse off than it would have been under the existing threshold IPER of $75,000?

Fewer new drugs reimbursed is a possible, not inevitable, outcome of a lowered maximum acceptable IPER. *Patients* who would otherwise have had subsidised access to these drugs will be worse off than would otherwise be the case, assuming the drugs that would otherwise have been listed all have clinically innovative value. However, the *population* could be better off under the lower threshold IPER of β_c even if some target patients are worse off. In other words, while some patients will be worse off, this loss of potential health effects will be outweighed by the health gain to patients who will be better off at the lower threshold IPER.[17] There are two reasons for this.

First, the possibility of a net reduction in the population's health is excluded under β_c but not under the historic maxWTP threshold IPER, which does not accommodate the effect of displacement. Second, as a consequence of using β_c rather than the maxWTP, the Institution has more information about the opportunities to correct the failure of the market to provide evidence of the aICER of unpatented programmes. This additional information might be obtained by allocating resources to developing this evidence rather than additional evidence of the maxWTP developed using population surveys. This additional information effectively expands the set of alternative strategies from which the best alternative strategy is selected. It makes it possible for the Institution to reallocate and improve the allocative efficiency of the health care budget. If there is no drug that has an IMER below β_c this does not mean that the rational Institution has no option available to improve the population's health within given resources—reallocation is that option.[18]

• How should the rational Institution respond to this threat?

The rational Institution should not respond to this threat by increasing the threshold IPER. The Institution should maintain β_c as the threshold IPER. It should also be prepared to accept that if the minimum acceptable IPER (to the Firms) of all new drugs is greater than β_c, then this is a signal to firms to improve their drug production processes and make clinical innovation more cost-effective. It is also a signal to the Institution to improve overall efficiency by reallocating across programmes rather than adopting new drugs.

---

[17] Who are these target patients who will be worse off? Until the drugs become available, there is no information about who these patients will be. This leads to the following situation. If we focus on the health benefit to the patients who will benefit from the new drug and not patients whose health is reduced because services are withdrawn to finance the drug, then we are saying that our value of the health gain for a patient is a function of the method by which it is produced, namely patented drugs, rather than say, unpatented respite care. One of the assumptions in the introduction to this book is that a universal access health care system will not have a preference for the method of producing a health gain. This assumption is revisited in Chap. 11.

[18] For a discussion of the possibility that the Institution will reject the drug but not reallocate, refer to the Conclusion to his book (Chap. 11).

8.9.2 Assumptions Revisited

The Game presented in this chapter made three important assumptions that influence both its results and their interpretation, however, these assumptions were not justified. These assumptions are addressed in more detail in subsequent chapters, and are summarised below.

The first assumption was that the marginal cost of production of the new drug was public information. In fact this information is typically private (known only to the firm). The resultant asymmetry in information can lead to the opportunity for additional strategies available to the firm which increase the chance that it can obtain a price at the previous higher threshold, despite the Reimburser lowering the threshold IPER. This issue is explored in more detail in Chaps. 9 and 10.

The second assumption made in this game was that the IPER of the new drug does not influence the Firm's R&D decisions and hence has no implications for the population's future health. The relationship between the IPER of the new drug and pharmaceutical R&D, and its implications for the decision to apply β_c as the threshold IPER, are explored in detail in Chaps. 9 and 10.

The third assumption is that there is no uncertainty in the value of any parameters. Clearly, there is uncertainty in all the parameters used in the GTM. The methods of characterising and analysing the uncertainty in the estimates of ΔC^P and $\overline{\Delta E^P}$ are well documented.[19] It is unlikely that any reasonable estimates of n, m and d exist. The implications of (1) uncertainty and absence of evidence of these parameters for PEA and (2) the use of β_c as the decision threshold, are discussed in more detail in the Conclusion to this book. However, at this stage it is useful to recognise the distinction between parameter uncertainty and absence of an incentive to develop evidence under the following two scenarios.

- An institution that uses economic evaluation and a maxWTP as a threshold provides an incentive for the market to develop estimates of ΔC^P and $\overline{\Delta E^P}$ and the associated uncertainty. It might also generate an incentive for academics to develop evidence of maxWTP. However, this situation provides no incentive to develop evidence of n, m and d. In particular, it does not address the market's failure to provide evidence of these parameters as they pertain to unpatented programmes. Nor are there any mechanisms analogous to new drug reimbursement within which this evidence has value in making a decision.

- An institution that places economic (decision) value on evidence of ΔC^P, $\overline{\Delta E^P}$, n, m and d by using β_c as a decision threshold and also addresses the failure of the market to provide this evidence will, in time, have estimates of these parameters with the associated uncertainty.

In summary, a critical difference between the application of β_c as a threshold IPER compared with other options is that it represents the first step in addressing the

---

[19] For example Willan and Briggs (2006).

market's failure to develop evidence of unpatented or unpatentable programmes and inputs. Hence is a first step towards providing the pharmaceutical industry with the price signal that the market would otherwise provide; the pharmaceutical industry's competition in the market for health effects from other ways of achieving these gains.

8.9.3 Economic Implications

From an economic perspective there are three additional implications of the results of this Game: (1) price is endogenous; (2) economic loss is underestimated by the conventional net benefit; and (3) thresholds above β_c introduce a potential economic loss and the existence of strategic behaviour leads us to predict that this economic loss will be maximised for any threshold above β_c.

8.9.3.1 Endogeneity of the Offer IPER

The new drug's offer IPER is endogenous to the reimbursement process, not exogenous as (necessarily) assumed in DTMs. Equilibrium price and offer price are both a function of the Reimburser's revealed threshold IPER. Therefore, while using a DTM is appropriate for estimating the ICER of a new drug and the associated uncertainty, it is not appropriate for the analysis of the decision to reimburse, which is a strategic situation. This endogeneity of price is entirely consistent with the US pharma-economic characterisation of cost-effectiveness analysis applied with a decision threshold of i (CEA_i) as price control: if the threshold price goes up, so does the price of new drugs. [This issue is discussed in detail in Pekarsky (2012, Appendix 7).] Health economists have also been aware of this issue since at least 1992 when the Australian Government started using economic evaluation for new drugs.[20] However, health economists do not appear to have considered the full impact of the endogeneity of input price where the manufacturer is a monopolist.

The impact on health economic thinking of recognising the endogeneity of price can be illustrated with the simple but instructive example of the idealised solution to the problem of revealing the shadow price of the budget constraint. The earliest example in health economics appears to be from Weinstein and Stason's 1977 paper on the foundations of CEA (Weinstein and Stason 1977) and the most recent from Weinstein's 2008 editorial on the imperative for the US to identify how much its citizens should be willing to pay per QALY gained (Weinstein 2008). Essentially,

---

[20] Consider Drummond's commentary on this scheme where he noted that a company needs to assume a price when it calculates an ICER and asks whether "the economic evaluation become an instrument for open price negotiation?" (Drummond 1992 p. 195)

the story involves the decision rule (threshold) being revealed by the actions of the Social Decision Maker. He ranks all programs by their ICER in ascending order and then continues allocating from this list until the budget is exhausted. The ICER of the last service is the decision rule; any new programmes with ICERs above this should be rejected and any with ICERs below this should be funded. Typically, the idealism of this particular solution to the problem of the shadow price of the budget constraint is attributed to the problems of interdependence between programmes, increasing and decreasing economies of scale, the vastness of the associated computational tasks and the disregard for equity by valuing all QALYs equally (Sendi et al. 2004; Weinstein 2008). Now introduce the possibility that firms price at exactly the revealed threshold, and that inputs that have prices below this and have market power increase their price. The budget that is initially exhausted will continue to grow, and this growth is the effect of the endogeneity of price and the public information about the revealed threshold.

8.9.3.2 The Conventionally Defined Net Benefit Underestimates the Economic Loss

If the historic threshold CEAi is greater than β_c $(i > \beta_c)$ then the economic loss associated with adoption at a given offer price, IPER $=f$, will be underestimated by the conventionally defined net benefit.

The proof is as follows:

Using the conventional method, the net benefit of reimbursement is:

$$NBm_i = i\Delta E^P - \Delta C^P = i\frac{\Delta C^P}{f_i} - \Delta C^P,$$

where f_i is the IPER of the new drug at the threshold i. Rearranging we have:

$$= \Delta C^P \left(\frac{i}{f_i} - 1 \right),$$

and dividing through by i we obtain the NBh$_i$ which is the conventional net benefit measured in health units and where the units are valued by i:

$$NBh_i = \Delta C^P \left(\frac{1}{f_i} - \frac{1}{i} \right).$$

However, as argued in Chap. 4 through 7, in order to assess the net economic benefit of the decision, we need to use β_c because this captures the competition in the health budget, including competition from strategies to improve reallocation. We use the net economic benefit (health) of reimbursement to illustrate this issue, although the same result is obtained by using the conventional net benefit with

$i = \beta_c$. We assess the net economic benefit of the new drug using the price that would occur had the threshold been i.

$$\text{NEBh}^R = \Delta E^P - \Delta E^D - \left(\Delta E^N - \Delta E^M\right) = \Delta C^P \left(\frac{1}{f_i} - \frac{1}{d} + \frac{1}{m} - \frac{1}{n}\right).$$

The underestimate of the economic loss of a threshold i is given by the difference in the two alternative measures of the net economic benefit:

$$\text{NBh}_i - \text{NEBh}^R = \Delta C^P \left(\frac{1}{f_i} - \frac{1}{i}\right) - \Delta C^P \left(\frac{1}{f_i} - \frac{1}{d} + \frac{1}{m} - \frac{1}{n}\right)$$
$$= \Delta C^P \left(\left(\frac{1}{n} - \frac{1}{m}\right) + \left(\frac{1}{d} - \frac{1}{i}\right)\right).$$

The underestimate of the net economic benefit that is a result of using the NBh_i as a proxy for net economic benefit increases:

- As the allocative inefficiency (m-n) increases;
- As the net population loss per additional health effect reimbursed at i ($i - d$) increases; and
- As the total additional expenditure, ΔC^P increases.

The underestimate of the economic loss as a consequence of using NBh_i as a proxy for economic loss rather than NEBh^R can also be expressed as:

$$\Delta C^P \left(\frac{1}{\beta_c} - \frac{1}{i}\right) \tag{8.3}$$

8.9.3.3 The Potential Maximum Economic Loss Is the Economic Loss

The non-strategic analyses in Chaps. 6 and 7 provide the metrics that allow us to calculate the potential economic loss in the case where a threshold is set too high and a new drug is approved at this threshold. There are three reasons why the actual loss is the predicted maximum potential loss possible from the strategy of reimbursement. First, for a given value of m, n and d, the maximum possible economic loss will be experienced on every drug sold at the higher than optimal threshold, i. The reason is that, under these givens, the size of the loss is determined by the additional cost of the new drug. The additional cost of the drug is a function of the price of each unit sold.

$$\Delta C^P = f_i \Delta E$$

The Game predicts that for each unit sold, the Firm will select the profit-maximising price, which is the threshold. Therefore, the maximum possible loss of using a threshold above β_c, which occurs when $f = i$, will be the economic loss that results from pricing above β_c at i.

Furthermore under the rules of the reimbursement game, which focus on the evidence of the incremental cost and effect as the rationale for an offer price, the Institution has no capacity to bargain below a revealed threshold IPER; only to regulate price down to that IPER. This situation further enforces the loss-maximising effect of an error in choosing a threshold. Finally this loss is experienced on more drugs than would have been be sold had the lower threshold price been enforced. These additional drugs will include drugs that are themselves more costly to manufacture, in terms of their IMER, than it costs for the health budget to produce health benefits from existing technologies, that is, the IMER $> \beta_c$.

8.9.4 Conclusion

This chapter's main conclusion is that the reimbursement process is more appropriately represented as a GTM rather than a DTM because the reimbursement process is strategic and new drug price is endogenous.

The main prediction from this game theoretic model is that a rational profit-maximising firm will price at the reimbursing institution's threshold IPER, whatever that price is. This prediction appears to be supported by the results of studies such as Devlin and Parkin (2004) that suggest that the majority of new drugs recommended by the UK NICE are priced close to or at the "inferred" or "implicit" threshold price.

Further evidence that firms price strategically is the quotation attributed to the CEO of Roche's pharmaceutical division and presented at the start of this chapter. Burns is quoted as saying of the higher price of the new drugs: "*the health economics holds up*". This position could be interpreted as follows: meeting the requirement of pricing at or below the institution's threshold IPER is the necessary and sufficient justification for its offer price.

The result of the game also leads to predictions about the consequences of lowering the threshold IPER.

First, we cannot assume that drugs that would otherwise be priced at the historic threshold IPER will no longer be made available at the lower threshold IPER. This result occurs because firms pricing at the higher price could be pricing above the marginal cost of production, hence they could still have an economic rent greater than or equal to zero at a lower price. However, the game theoretic structure of this model also introduces the possibility that firms can use information asymmetry (private information about the marginal costs of production) to lobby for an above-threshold price for a new drug. This possibility is explored in more detail in Chaps. 9 and 10.

Second, the population will always be better off with a threshold IPER of β_c, because the following two situations are avoided:

- The net effect of reimbursement on the population's health is negative $(d < f)$; and
- The best alternative strategy to reimbursement at the offer IPER is not implemented.

The use of d as the decision threshold rather than $k(>d)$ avoids the first but not the second situation.

Finally, we can conclude that GTMs characterise and accommodate the endogeneity of price, whereas DTMs do not. For example, if the optimality of disinvestment increases and d is used as the threshold, then DTMs would lead us to predict that the loss associated with reimbursement decisions is decreasing because the net effect of adoption and displacement is more likely to be positive. However, as $d \rightarrow m > d$ then if $i = d$, i is increasing and hence β_c increases. From Eq. (8.3) we see that this will in turn increase the economic loss associated with adoption decisions, because firms are predicted to price at the increasing i. Therefore only GTMs correctly predict that the economic loss will increase as the suboptimality of displacement is reduced and hence i increases.

The Reimburser is satisfied that the population's health will not be worse off as a consequence of selecting β_c rather than k. This is the case even though some patients might be worse off at the lower threshold price. However, the Reimburser remains uncomfortable with the following three explicit assumptions made in the model:

- Evidence of the IMER is in the public domain;
- There is no relationship between the IPER and future innovation; and
- There is no uncertainty in the value of β_c.

She is particularly concerned with the second of these assumptions. This assumption is consistent with claims made by pharma-economists Jena and Philipson (2008) in their support for the case for the Firm's Preferred Price (the FPP). These authors argue that a decision threshold that is based on maximising health from existing technologies does not capture the dynamic welfare implications of this relationship between price and future health.

The previous chapters described the derivation of β_c and it is true that it explicitly excludes any consideration of the relationship between the IPER and the future health of the population that is the result of innovation. It is clear that the evidence base developed so far, while it identifies a threshold IPER suitable for the economic context of her budget, does not inform the Reimburser on the critical question she has identified from the reframed political economy presented in Chap. 1:

- How should the Institution respond to the threat from Pharma that reducing the price below the FPP will result in the future population's health being worse that otherwise would be the case?

The next step in developing the evidence to inform the Reimburser's response to the main Pharma threat would appear to be to compare the payoff with the population's health of selecting β_c as the decision threshold compared with the payoff of choosing the FPP. But what is the FPP? What are its theoretical underpinnings? How does the FPP capture information about the relationship between price and innovation? Does it capture information about the economic context in the same way that β_c does?

The Reimburser requests that her Health Economic Adviser prepare a report on this issue which is provided in Pekarsky (2012, Appendix 7).

References

Antonanzas F, Juarez-Castello C, Rodriguez-Ibeas R (2011) Should health authorities offer risk-sharing contracts to pharmaceutical firms? A theoretical approach. Health Econ Policy Law 6 (3):391–403. doi:10.1017/S1744133111000016

Berenson A (2006) A cancer drug shows promise, at a price that many can't pay. New York Times, February 15

Boggild M, Palace J, Barton P, Ben-Shlomo Y, Bregenzer T, Dobson C, Gray R (2009) Multiple sclerosis risk sharing scheme: two year results of clinical cohort study with historical comparator. Br Med J 339:b4677. doi:10.1136/bmj.b4677

Culyer A, McCabe C, Briggs A, Claxton K, Buxton M, Akehurst R, Sculpher M, Brazier J (2007) Searching for a threshold, not setting one: the role of the National Institute for Health and Clinical Excellence. J Health Serv Res Policy 12(1):56–58. doi:10.1258/135581907779497567

Devlin N, Parkin D (2004) Does NICE have a cost-effectiveness threshold and what other factors influence its decisions? A binary choice analysis. Health Econ 13(5):437–452. doi:10.1002/hec.864

Drummond MF (1992) Basing prescription drug payment on economic analysis: the case of Australia. Health Aff 11

Elshaug A, Hiller J, Tunis S, Moss J (2007) Challenges in Australian policy processes for disinvestment from existing, ineffective health care practices. Aust New Zealand Health Policy 4(23)

Garber A, Skinner J (2008) Is American health care uniquely inefficient? J Econ Perspect 22 (4):27–50

Grüne-Yanoff T, Schweinzer P (2008) The roles of stories in applying game theory. J Econ Methodol 15(2):131–146

Jena AB, Philipson TJ (2008) Cost-effectiveness analysis and innovation. J Health Econ 27:1224–1236

Landsburg S (1988) Price theory and applications. The Dreyden Press, Chicago, IL

Mansley EC, Elbasha EH, Teutsch SM, Berger ML (2007) The decision to conduct a head-to-head comparative trial: a game-theoretic analysis. Med Decis Mak 27(4):364–379. doi:10.1177/0272989x07303825

Pearson S, Littlejohns P (2007) Reallocating resources: how should the National Institute for Health and Clinical Excellence guide disinvestment efforts in the National Health Service? J Health Serv Res Policy 12(3):160–165. doi:10.1258/135581907781542987

Pekarsky BAK (2012) Trust, constraints and the counterfactual: reframing the political economy of new drug price. Dissertation, University of Adelaide http://digital.library.adelaide.edu.au/dspace/handle/2440/79171. Accessed 25 Dec 2013

Sendi P, Al MJ, Gafni A, Birch S (2004) Portfolio theory and the alternative decision rule of cost-effectiveness analysis: theoretical and practical considerations. Soc Sci Med 58 (10):1853–1855. doi:10.1016/j.socscimed.2004.10.001

Watson J (2002) Strategy: an introduction to game theory. W. W. Norton and Company, New York

Weinstein MC (2008) How much are Americans willing to pay for a quality-adjusted life year?
    Med Care 46(4):343–345
Weinstein MC, Stason WB (1977) Foundations of cost-effectiveness analysis for health and
    medical practices. N Engl J Med 296(13):716–721
Willan A, Briggs A (2006) The statistical analysis of cost-effectiveness data. Wiley, Chichester
Wright D (2004) The drug bargaining pharmaceutical regulation in Australia. J Health Econ
    23:785–813

Part III
The New Drug Decision Threshold and the Relationship Between Price and Innovation

Chapter 9
The "Pharmaceutical R&D Financing" Game

Abstract This chapter presents "The pharmaceutical R&D financing" game in which the Institution lowers the decision threshold and must respond to a pharmaceutical industry Threat. Firms claim that the capital market fails to provide funds for pharmaceutical Research and Development (R&D); it is a risky investment and returns are long-term. Hence, firms finance R&D through internal funds generated by above marginal cost pricing of drugs. If institutions use monopsonist power to bargain down prices, there will be insufficient funds to finance the R&D that society requires. The population will be worse off. This claim leads to the following paradox: *Why should the health budget finance pharmaceutical R&D without a formal contractual arrangement if firms and pharma-economists are claiming that the capital markets are unwilling to take on this risk, even with the protection of legally enforceable contracts?* The Game is structured as a choice by firms between the two strategies to raise funds: Lobby (approach the Institution to increase prices) or Borrow (go to the capital market). I conclude that there is no incentive for the Institution to finance pharmaceutical R&D through higher prices, unless a contract is negotiated. However, in this case, if institutions are more risk adverse than banks, this strategy (Lobby with Contract) will be more expensive for firms than approaching the capital market. The practice by firms of financing most of their investment in R&D from internal funds is more likely to be the result of these internal funds being imperfectly priced by institutions, not failure in the capital market.

9.1 The Reimburser's Problem

A Firm approaches the Reimburser with a new drug and evidence of its additional cost, ΔC^P, and effect, $\overline{\Delta E^P}$. This new drug is substantially more effective than the best available existing therapy $\left(\overline{\Delta E^P} \gg 0 \right)$. The Firm's offer IPER, f, is much higher than the health shadow price ($f \gg \beta_c$). These two conditions mean that the drug's reimbursement will have a significant budgetary impact, in this case:

© Springer International Publishing Switzerland 2015

B.A.K. Pekarsky, *The New Drug Reimbursement Game*,

DOI 10.1007/978-3-319-08903-4_9

$$f \overline{\Delta E^p} \sim 5\% B^P,$$

where B^P is the drug budget. Existing non-drug programmes with an aICER of d will need to be displaced to provide the funds from a fixed health budget to finance the new drug. These programmes are unpatented, non-pharmaceutical programmes such as respite care and free dental services. The budget is currently economically efficient ($n = m$) and displacement is optimal ($d = m$) therefore:

$$\beta_c = m$$

The Firm argues that an IPER of f, where $f > \beta_c$, will ensure that there are sufficient internal funds to finance the development of a future drug. The Firm claims that it will invest the entire premium over β_c into new drug R&D. This investment is an amount $\overline{\mathcal{R}}$ where:

$$\overline{\mathcal{R}} = \overline{\Delta E^p}(f - \beta_c).$$

The Firm argues that it needs to fund R&D from internal funds because the capital market fails to finance pharmaceutical R&D; even with formal contracts, the investment is too risky and the returns, if they occur, are too long-term. The Firm supports this argument with peer reviewed papers and US government reports that state that capital market imperfection limits pharmaceutical firms' access to external funds and hence firms rely on internal funds generated from additional profit from higher prices (Vernon 2003; International Trade Administration 2004; Santerre and Vernon 2006). These authors conclude that without funds from economic rent there will not be enough funds available to finance the R&D that society requires. Therefore, lower prices, which will reduce the amount of economic rent and hence internal funds, are not in the long-term interest of consumers. The Firm's case for financing pharmaceutical R&D using funds sourced from higher prices appears strong.

The Firm also provides the Reimburser with a US Congressional Budget Office Report (2006) that refers to Reinhardt (2001)[1] in which the Report's authors write that:

> A relatively close relationship exists between drug firms' current R&D spending and current sales revenue for two reasons. First, successful new drugs generate large cash flows that can be invested in R&D (their manufacturing costs are usually very low relative to their price). Second, alternative sources of investment capital—from the bond and stock markets—are not perfect substitutes for cash flow financing. Those alternative sources of capital are more expensive because lenders and prospective new shareholders require compensation (in the form of higher returns) for the additional risk they bear compared with the firm, which has more information about the drug under development, its current status, and its ultimate chance of success. (p. 9)

---

[1] Whether the authors convey Reinhardt's intent is unclear to me.

The Firm uses this statement to lend support to their argument that if the Firm is required to go to the Capital Market to finance its R&D, it will be more costly and the price of future new drugs will need to be increased to compensate for this.

The Reimburser is confused. What does it mean to say that the Firm *"has more information about the drug under development, its current status, and its ultimate chance of success"*? What sort of information do companies have prior to conducting an RCT? What information do they have that is not understood by the Capital Market? Can this information be provided to and understood by Institutions? The Reimburser is reminded of a paper she read recently on the benefits of risk-sharing arrangements for pharmaceuticals and the economics of warranties where the authors describe warranties as a method of signalling high quality when it is not observable and the costs of measuring that quality are high (Cook et al. 2008, p. 555).

The Reimburse asks: "What are these unobservable aspects of quality? What is this information firms have and why would they not put it in the public domain? How are they going to obtain this information without costly RCTs?"

The US literature does provide alternative explanations for why large pharmaceutical firms use internal funds. Hall (2002) identified a number of possible reasons, including information asymmetry, moral hazard on the part of firms and a preference by the capital market for collateral in the form of physical assets. She concludes that there is a possible case for government subsidies for smaller (start-up) firms. Hall also concludes that it is hard to establish any evidence of a "financing gap" for large established firms, but that it is possible to identify a preference for internal funding (Hall 2002 p. 49).

The Reimburser recognises that there could be an alternative explanation for the observation that firms finance R&D from internal funds. She hypothesises that firms prefer to finance through internal funds (financed by economic rent) because this method is cheaper than raising funds through the capital market. It is cheaper because, unlike the capital market, the Reimburser does not require firms to present a case for financing the NME's R&D, nor does it require the firm to agree to a contract that sets out the capital repayments and interest payments.[2]

Financing pharmaceutical R&D from the health budget comes at a tangible and significant cost to the population's health today. The Reimburser reviews the proposed budget cuts for programmes over the next 3 financial years as the whole of government responds to the increasing pressure of government debt. In this climate, services that are no less cost-effective that the new drug will need to be displaced to finance the pharmaceutical R&D premium. This displacement occurs

---

[2] For example, the previous quotation from the Congressional Budget Office Report notes that internal funds are a cheaper source of funds than the capital market because this market requires compensation for the additional risk they bear in relation to the firm because the firm has more information about the drug being developed. However, the authors do not clarify why the providers of these internal funds, purchasers and public research funding organisations, do not require this compensation. This is the case even though the authors identify higher drug prices as a source of these funds.

in addition to the displacement to finance the additional costs of the health effects from the new drug. Furthermore, there is no contractual arrangement with the Firm to guarantee a return to consumers on their risky investment: their own health today foregone to increase the population's health tomorrow.

The Reimburser wonders how risky it is to use the health budget to finance pharmaceutical R&D and whether her population can bear this risk. After all, firms claim that the capital market finds it too risky to lend to firms, and unlike the Reimburser, the capital market is protected by a contract.

The Reimburser asks:

- How should the rational and risk-averse or risk-neutral Institution respond to the Threat?

9.2   The Pharmaceutical R&D Financing Game

We use a game theoretic model to identify the underlying strategies and payoffs in the Pharmaceutical R&D Financing Game. The Game is then used to make a number of predictions that are tested against real world observations and identify the conditions required for the risk-averse Institution to respond to this threat by increasing the threshold price above β_c. Finally we consider whether, if these conditions are met, the Firm will continue to have a preference for funding R&D from internal funds rather than the capital market.

An adaption of Grüne-Yanoff and Schweinzer's Architecture of Game Theory (Grüne-Yanoff and Schweinzer 2008) is used to develop the story as an applied game. This framework comprises the following elements (1) World (the economic problem); (2) Game, which comprises the narrative and the game structure; and (3) Theory Proper. This framework is detailed in Chaps. 2 and 6 and Pekarsky (2012, Appendix 1). The following three Sects. (9.3, 9.4 and 9.5) set out these components, and then the solution is presented in Sect. 9.6.

9.3   World (The Economic Problem)

Firms use internal funds rather than the capital market to finance pharmaceutical R&D. This is because internal funds are less costly than capital market funds due to imperfections in the capital market, identified by authors such as Santerre and Vernon (2006). These imperfections are a consequence of the capital market being unable to incorporate the full long-term benefits to society of investments in pharmaceutical R&D. They are also a consequence of information asymmetry; according to a US Congressional Report (2006), firms have information about the future benefits of a drug that is not available to capital markets or is costly to make available. Firms use the evidence of funding preferences and the associated economic rationale sourced from the peer reviewed literature to provide an evidence base for the following threat:

> The FPP is the price that is necessary in order to ensure that sufficient R&D is available for the future. If prices are lower, then funds will need to be sourced from the capital market rather than internal funds. This will increase the costs of capital and combined with the lower prices, will mean that firms will reduce investments in R&D and hence there will be fewer new drugs in the future and the population will be worse off.
>
> • How should the rational Institution respond to this threat?

9.4 Model

The Model comprises the Narrative and the Game Structure.

9.4.1 Narrative

The Game starts when the Firm decides whether to raise the funds for R&D from either the health budget (Lobby) or capital market (Borrow). The Firm also has the option to do Nothing.

9.4.1.1 Lobby

The Firm's first option is Lobby (L): lobby purchasers to pay higher prices for the existing drug. This lobbying process uses various submissions, reports and delegations to influence decisions that impact the price of a new drug and hence the profit for a given quantity of the new drug sold. The Lobbyists' key claim is that purchasers must not use their monopsony powers to negotiate prices below the offer price because if this occurs there will be insufficient funds available to finance the R&D required for future drugs. The Lobbyists' position can be summarised as: *only economic rent can finance R&D efficiently, and reduced economic rent means proportionally less R&D and less R&D means fewer new drugs and hence less health in the future.*

The Institution can either reject or accept the Firm's lobbying. If it rejects the lobbying, the game ends. If the lobbying is successful, a higher price for the existing drug is agreed upon and the additional economic profit that results from this lobbying provides additional internal funds that are invested in NME R&D.

These additional funds are sourced by the higher prices on existing drugs, which are in turn financed from the fixed health budget by displacing existing services that have an aICER of d. These services are the least cost-effective of existing services (displacement is optimal). The budget is currently economically efficient; there are no alternative ways of producing health within existing technologies and resources that will improve health for the population.[3] Therefore, because the conditions of optimality of displacement, $d = m$, and economic efficiency, $m = n$, are met and the budget is fixed, we conclude that $\beta_c = m$.

The Firm's investment in pharmaceutical R&D might or might not result in an NME; there is a risk. This risk is characterised inconsistently in the literature.[4] However, the claim by the Lobbyists is that this risk is so high and the return, if it occurs, is so far into the future that the capital market will not finance this R&D, or alternatively, will finance this R&D at prohibitively high rates. In the context of this model, this risk is simply expressed as a probability, q, that an NME of a given value of clinical innovation will be brought to the market and a probability $(1 - q)$ that there will be no NME brought to the market as a consequence of the Firm's decision to invest in new drug R&D.

If the R&D is not successful, the Game ends and there are no mechanisms in place for the Institution's investment to be returned, so there is a loss to the Institution equivalent to its original investment. If the R&D is successful then the Firm selects an offer price for the future drug and the Institution can choose to reimburse the future drug at the offer price or do nothing. (The details of this part of this Game are addressed in Game 1 Sect. 8.6.1.1.)

9.4.1.2 Borrow

The second R&D financing option available to the Firm is Borrow (B): go to the Capital Market and attempt to borrow all the funds required for the development of an NME. The process of borrowing to finance the costs of a specific project requires the Firm to present a Bank with evidence of its financial status, the funds it requires, and the likely success of its investment in terms of future revenue and profit. This estimate of future profit would need to include an assumption about the future revenue from the future drug, which would in turn require assumptions about: the potential clinical innovation of the future drug, $\overline{\Delta E^p}$; the estimated costs of producing the additional health effects (the IMER, in this case c per QALY); the

---

[3] There are ways to improve the health of groups of patient groups using technologies not currently financed. However, the additional cost of financing these technologies will require services to be displaced and health effects lost. The net effect of the loss from displacement and gain for the patient group will be to reduce the population's health because the new technologies are less cost-effective than the least cost-effective of existing technologies.

[4] A discussion of two ways that the pharma-economic literature and Pharma characterise and quantify risk and additional sources of variation in firm profits is presented in Pekarsky (2012, Appendix 8).

market share of the future drug; the future threshold price; and the IPER of the future drug.

We assume that if the R&D is unsuccessful then there is no repayment of the loan. This assumption is a simplification but it is consistent with the observation that there is limited physical collateral held by the pharmaceutical Firm and that this is a factor influencing the decision by the Capital Market to lend to Firms. It also allows the riskiness of the loan to be characterised as part of the payoff to the Capital Market.[5]

The Bank (a lender in the Capital Market) will review the case presented by the Firm and solve for the Bank's minimum acceptable interest rate. The Bank's choice of offer price (interest rate), θ, will also be influenced by its assessment of the Firm's maximum acceptable price. We assume the Bank selects an offer price of θ. The Firm can either reject or accept the Bank's proposal to lend at a rate θ, or it may enter into a negotiation if its maximum acceptable interest rate is higher than the Bank's minimum acceptable rate. If the Firm and the Bank agree on an interest rate, the Firm will Borrow an amount, $\mathcal{R}$, with a requirement that it pays an interest rate of θ, as well as repaying the loan from the revenue from the future drug, should the R&D be successful. A contractual arrangement ensures repayment if there is success and sets out the shared understanding of the risks associated with the loan. If there is no success, there will be no repayment. This condition, which is set out in the contract, makes the loan "high risk". It characterises the claimed failure of the Capital Market to finance this R&D due to high risk.

The Bank has a second option; lend to a risk-free borrower at a rate of τ, therefore its payoff from lending to the Firm is net of the opportunity cost of this foregone activity. This use of an economic payoff for the Bank is consistent with the use of an economic payoff for both the Firm and the Institution.

If the R&D is successful, the Firm will offer the NME to the Institution at an IPER $= f$. The Institution will either reimburse the future drug at this price or do nothing. If it rejects the drug at this price, then the Game ends. There will be no repayment to the Bank because there is no revenue stream associated with the future drug, despite the success of the R&D in bringing a drug to market.

---

[5] This problem uses the terms "investment" for the Institution and "loan" for the funding from the Capital Market. The use of the term "investment" highlights that there is an expected dividend if the R&D is successful. The use of the term "loan" suggests a schedule of repayments of the capital with an agreed interest payment. It is unrealistic to assume that the Capital Market will have no capital returned from its loan in the event of a failed R&D; this would mean the Firm becomes bankrupt. However, this device, assuming that there is no return to the Capital Market on its loan if R&D is unsuccessful, allows the claimed riskiness of this loan to be characterized and also simplifies the math. The critical issue is that the Firm enters a formal agreement with the Capital Market that ensures an agreed payment if it is successful and there is no such agreement with the Institution and the dividend is instead a future drug, which the Institution needs to pay for.

9.4.1.3   Some Other Parts to the Story

We assume that the expected incremental effect of the drug, $\overline{\Delta E^p}$, is independent of the method used to finance the future drug. The probability of success (q) or failure $(1 - q)$ of the R&D process is also assumed to be independent of the method used to finance the R&D for the future drug. While the Firm would need to present a business case to the Bank to support its application for a loan, it is assumed that no such documentation is required if the Firm chooses to lobby the Institution to obtain these funds. And while the Firm is required to repay the loan and pay interest to the Bank if there is success, it is not required to make such payments to an Institution if the R&D is successful.

The relationships between the additional cost, additional effect and IPER compared with the best existing drug are detailed in Game 1, Sect. 8.6.1.1. For example, the IPER of the new drug is assumed to be the result of a higher price for the new drug, and no additional savings elsewhere in the health budget are expected.

9.4.1.4   The Rules of Engagement

1. If the Institution is indifferent between reimbursing that drug at the offer price and the best alternative action then the Institution must accept the Firm's offer price for the future drug.
2. The Institution cannot negotiate below the offer price if the offer price is at or below the decision threshold.

9.4.1.5   The Threat

The FPP is the price that is necessary in order to ensure that sufficient R&D is available for the future. If prices are lower, then capital funds will need to be sourced from the capital market rather than internal funds. This situation will increase the costs of capital and combined with the lower prices, firms will reduce investments in R&D and hence there will be fewer new drugs in the future and the population will be worse off.

9.4.2   The Game Structure

Game 2 is presented in extensive form as a dynamic game (there is a sequence of decisions) of incomplete information (there is uncertainty in the payoff to R&D, but not in the probabilities of success and fail) and no private information (all information that is certain is in the public domain, including the value of the probability of success or ail of R&D). Even though the process of raising R&D funds, developing new drugs and obtaining reimbursement occurs over a period of several years, the Game is represented as occurring in one period. This simpler specification allows the key strategic incentives to be identified. In Chap. 10 the findings from Games 1 and 2 inform a three-period game of the drug R&D process; Game 3.

9.4.2.1 Extensive Form Representation of the Game

The extensive form representation of the Game is presented in Fig. 9.1.

9.4.2.2 Players, Actions and Payoffs

There are three players: the Firm (F), the Institution (I) and the Capital Market (C). The payoffs in the Game are listed in that order in Fig. 9.1.

Game 2 starts when the Firm approaches either the Capital Market or the Institution to raise the funds required to develop an NME. The Game in Fig. 9.1 sets out three actions available to the Firm in the first stage: do Nothing (N), Lobby (L) or Borrow (B). The details associated with each action follow.

Firm Chooses to Do Nothing (N)

If the Firm chooses to do Nothing, the Game ends and the payoff to each player is zero. The players will all continue to make profits (F and C) or health gains for the population (I) from existing activities, the outcomes of which are assumed not to be impacted by this particular Game.

Firm Chooses to Lobby (L)

Lobbying (L) involves the Firm making a case to the Institution that it should provide the research funds $\overline{\mathcal{R}}$ via higher prices on the existing drug. If the Firm chooses to Lobby (L) the Institution, the Institution can choose to either Accept (A) or do Nothing (N) in response to the proposal by the Firm to raise additional funds through internal revenue (economic rent) on the existing drug. If the Institution chooses to do Nothing (N) in response to the Lobbying (L), the Game ends and the payoff to each of the Firm, the Institution and the Capital Market is zero.

If the Institution chooses to Accept (A) the Lobbying (L) and pay the Firm the additional economic rent, $\overline{\mathcal{R}}$ per unit sold, the Firm will invest the entire funds[6] into

---

[6] In fact the evidence suggests that the Firm will invest <33 % into R&D for new drugs (see Vernon's Equation (International Trade Administration 2004 p. 29). Reinhardt also makes this point, although indicates the percentage of revenue rather than economic rent that goes to R&D (Reinhardt 2007 pp. 41–43). The implications of relaxing this assumption are considered in the discussion.

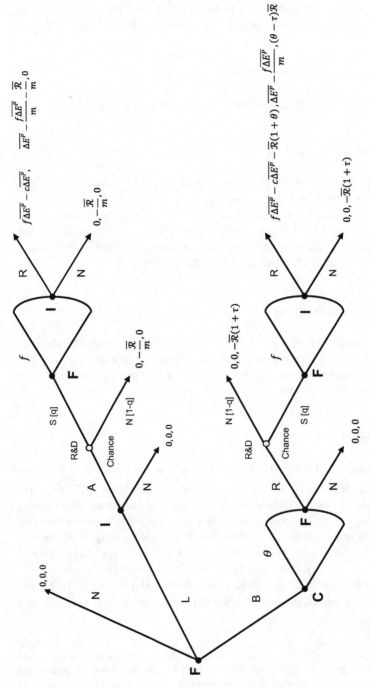

Fig. 9.1 The pharmaceutical R&D financing game

the R&D and the result will be either Success (S), an NME, or No success (N), no new drug. The probability of these two outcomes is q and $1 - q$ respectively. If there is No success (N) the game stops and the payoffs to the Firm and the Capital Market are both zero, whereas the financial payoff to the Institution is the net financial cost for the population's health budget: $-\overline{\mathcal{R}}$

The payoff to the Institution is the loss of the Institution's investment of health budget funds into the R&D process raised via the increased price of existing drugs paid to the Firm as a consequence of lobbying. The health payoff to the Institution if there is No success (N) is the net change in the population's health:

$$\Delta E = -\frac{\overline{\mathcal{R}}}{m}.$$

The payoff is the loss in health effects as a consequence of financing the pharmaceutical R&D by displacing services with an aICER of m. The health budget is currently economically efficient and displacement is optimal ($d = m$) therefore the NEBh (which is negative) is the same as the net health loss for the population.

If the R&D is successful, then the Firm will offer the future NME at an IPER of f. The Institution will either Reimburse (R) or do Nothing (N) when the Firm presents the future drug at the offer price of f. If the Institution Reimburses (R) the drug at the offer price, the payoff to the Firm, π_F is:

$$\pi_F = f\overline{\Delta E^p} - c\overline{\Delta E^p} + \overline{\mathcal{R}} - \overline{\mathcal{R}} = \overline{\Delta E^p}(f - c).$$

This payoff comprises:

- The revenue from the new drug that has an IPER f where the total additional health effects for the target patients are $\overline{\Delta E^p}$ and hence revenue is $f\overline{\Delta E^p}$;
- Less the costs of production of the future drug, an IMER of c per unit additional health effect produced ($\overline{\Delta E^p}$) and hence a total manufacturing cost of $c\overline{\Delta E^p}$;
- Plus the amount raised by lobbying, $\overline{\mathcal{R}}$; and
- Less the investment into NME R&D, $\overline{\mathcal{R}}$.

The Lobbying is assumed to be costless; an assumption that is relaxed in the discussion.

The payoff to the Capital Market will be zero and the payoff to the Institution, the net health benefit to the population, ΔE will be:

$$\Delta E = \overline{\Delta E^p} - \frac{f\overline{\Delta E^p}}{m} - \frac{\overline{\mathcal{R}}}{m}.$$

This payoff comprises:

- $$\overline{\Delta E^p}$$

– The additional health effects of the future new drug for target patients, compared with the best existing therapy in the future;

•

$$\frac{f \overline{\Delta E^p}}{m}$$

– The health effects lost due to the requirement to displace an amount $f\overline{\Delta E^p}$ of services with aICER $= m$ to finance the future drug; and

•

$$\frac{\mathcal{R}}{m}$$

– The health effects displaced to finance the additional amount $\overline{\mathcal{R}}$.

If the Institution chooses to Not reimburse (N) the future NME at the offer price, the payoff to the Firm and the Bank is zero and the payoff to the Institution is the incremental change in the population's health:

$$\Delta E = -\frac{\mathcal{R}}{m}.$$

This payoff is the loss to the Institution from displacing services at an aICER of m to finance the amount lobbied for by the Firm, $\overline{\mathcal{R}}$.

Firm Chooses to Borrow (B)

If the Firm chooses to Borrow (B) and accepts the Capital Market's offer price of θ, it borrows the funds and if the R&D is successful and the Institution agrees to the offer price, the Firm's payoff to Borrow (B) is:

$$\pi_F = f\overline{\Delta E^p} - c\overline{\Delta E^p} - \overline{\mathcal{R}}(1+\theta) = \overline{\Delta E^p}(f - c) - \overline{\mathcal{R}}(1+\theta).$$

This payoff (π_F) differs from the payoff of the strategy Lobby followed by Successful R&D and Reimbursement of the future drug, by the amount that the Firm is required to repay for the loan from the Capital Market, an amount of:

$$\overline{\mathcal{R}}(1+\theta).$$

The Institution's expected payoff to this series of eventualities is the change in the population's health:

$$\Delta E = \overline{\Delta E^p} - \frac{f\overline{\Delta E^p}}{m}.$$

This payoff comprises:

•
$$\overline{\Delta E^P}$$

- The additional health effects of the future new drug compared to the best existing therapy in the future, and

•
$$\frac{f\overline{\Delta E^P}}{m}$$

- The health effects lost due to the requirement to displace an amount $f\overline{\Delta E^P}$ of services with aICER m to finance the future drug.

And the Capital Market's payoff is:

$$\pi_C = \theta\overline{\mathcal{R}} - \tau\overline{\mathcal{R}} = \overline{\mathcal{R}}(\theta - \tau),$$

where $\theta\overline{\mathcal{R}}$ is the interest from the loan to the Firm and $\tau\overline{\mathcal{R}}$ is the foregone interest from a loan that the Capital Market could have made by lending to a zero-risk borrower.

If the Firm does not accept the Capital Market's offer of funds at price θ then the Game ends and there is a payoff of zero for each player. If the Firm agrees to the Capital Market's offer of i and the R&D is unsuccessful then the Game ends and the payoff to the Capital Market is a loss of:

$$\overline{\mathcal{R}}(1 + \tau).$$

The loss of $\overline{\mathcal{R}}(1 + \tau)$ includes the economic loss (the foregone interest), as well as the loss of the capital loaned to the Firm. In simple terms, if the Bank had instead lent to the risk-free borrower, it would have retained the capital and received the interest.

The payoff to the Firm is zero.

If the Capital Market lends to the Firm and the R&D is successful and the Institution does not accept the offer price, f, then the payoffs are a loss of $\overline{\mathcal{R}}(1 + \tau)$ and zero for the Capital Market and the Firm, respectively.[7]

---

[7] The Institution and Firm can of course enter a bargaining process. However, the key issue is that the public domain decision threshold combined with the requirement for the Institution to agree to reimburse the new drug if its price per effect is less than or equal to the threshold means that the profit maximizing offer price. If it cannot offer the drug at this price then it will be able to assess the impact of this constraint via the backward induction process. This situation is illustrated in Game 1, Chap. 8.

9.4.2.3   Parameters and variables

- $\overline{\mathcal{R}}$ is the Firm's fixed cost for developing and trialling a future drug.
- q is the probability that the R&D will be successful and result in a future drug.
- $\overline{\Delta E^p}$ is the additional health effect of the future drug (should R&D be successful) compared with the best alternative therapy at the time.
- m is the aICER of services displaced in order to finance the additional cost of existing drug that is necessary to raise the funds for pharmaceutical R&D. It is also the aICER of the services displaced to finance additional cost of the future drug.
- c is the IMER, the additional cost per unit of additional health effect of manufacturing the future drug, compared to current drug.
- f is the IPER of the future drug.
- θ is the interest rate charged by the Capital Market to the Firm, over the period of the loan.
- τ is the interest rate charged by the Capital Market to a zero-risk borrower.

The parameters and variables that describe the payoffs of the actions available to the Institution can be specified in terms of the total cost and unit cost of achieving them.

- $$\frac{f \overline{\Delta E^p}}{m}$$

  - is the health effects displaced if the additional cost of the additional health gains from the future drug $\left(f \overline{\Delta E^p} \right)$ are financed by displacing services of an aICER m.

- $$\frac{\overline{\mathcal{R}}}{m}$$

  - is the health effects displaced if the additional costs of financing firm R&D $\left(\overline{\mathcal{R}} \right)$ are financed by displacing services of an aICER m.

9.4.2.4   Conditions

- The value of q, the probability of success of R&D, is known, even though the *ex-ante* outcome of R&D is uncertain. There is no uncertainty in the value of any other parameters or variables in the Game at any stage in the Game for either player.

- There is no private information, for example, the costs of manufacturing are known by all players.
- The Institution is risk-averse or risk-neutral.
- The Capital Market is risk-neutral.
- The Firm is efficient in its R&D process; there is no way of trialling and developing a future drug that would reduce the fixed costs of R&D.
- There is no option for the Institution or another Firm to invest in the development of a non-pharmaceutical innovation, such as a new medical device. The implications of relaxing this assumption are considered in the discussion.

- $$\overline{\Delta E^p} > 0.$$

  - The future drug brought to the Institution is clinically innovative, that is, it has a clinical advantage compared with the best available existing therapy for the target group of patients. It is constant for the identified group of target patients, and is known with certainty.

- $$m > 0.$$

  - The aICER of services displaced to finance the additional financial costs of the future drug is greater than zero. It is also the least cost-effective of all existing options to contract programmes (efficient displacement). Using PEA terminology: $d = m = \beta_c$.

- $$\frac{\overline{\Delta E^p}}{m}, \frac{\overline{\mathcal{R}}}{m} > 0.$$

  - It follows from $\overline{\Delta E^p}$, $\overline{\mathcal{R}}$, $m > 0$ that displacing services to finance the additional costs of the pharmaceutical R&D and the future drug will lead to a loss in health effects for patients who would otherwise have received these services.

- $$f \geq 0$$

  - The IPER of the future drug compared to the best available therapy is greater than or equal to 0.

- $$c > 0$$

  - The IMER is greater than zero.

- $$0 > \theta, \tau, q > 1$$

  - The interest rates and the probability of success of R&D all lie between 0 and 1.

9.4.2.5   And Other Assumptions

1. It is assumed that both lobbying and preparation of a business case for the Capital Market are costless. This assumption is not consistent with the real world experience and the implications of relaxing this are considered in the discussion.
2. The costs of R&D, the incremental effect of the NME and cost of its production are independent of the method used to finance the R&D.
3. The health budget is fixed.
4. The health budget is initially economically efficient ($m = n$)and the displacement process is optimal ($m = d$). Therefore the quantitative value of the health shadow price β_c is m.
5. Because the health budget is economically efficient and displacement is optimal, the net economic benefit or loss of reimbursement is the same as the net health benefit or loss for the population.
6. If the Institution is indifferent between reimbursing a drug at the offer price and doing nothing it must reimburse the drug.
7. Both the Firm and Capital Market seek to maximise economic rent.
8. The Institution seeks to maximise npvPH from allocations and purchases made from this and future budgets.
9. The Firm allocates the entire economic rent raised through lobbying into the R&D process for new drugs. The implications of relaxing this assumption are explored in the discussion.

9.5   Theory Proper

The Game draws upon the following theory: a player will select from options so as to maximise the expected economic profit or the expected economic value of the health effect. The latter is the same as maximising the population health effect because the budget is economically efficient (see Chap. 7). The solution concept used for the Game is Backward Induction.

9.6   Solution

The key strategic choice is whether the Firm chooses to Lobby, Borrow or do Nothing at the start of the Game. We compare the expected payoff to the Firm for these three actions by considering the consequences of each initial decision. These eventualities are in turn influenced by both the results of the chance nodes (the chance result of R&D) and the strategic response by the other players. We solve the Game by backward induction, starting with the outcome had the Firm chosen to Lobby in Stage 1.

9.6.1 Lobby

9.6.1.1 Stage 5 (Lobby): The Decision by the Institution to Reimburse the Future Drug at the Offer Price or Do Nothing

The process of displacement is optimal and the budget is allocatively and technically efficient, hence:

$$\beta_c = m.$$

Therefore the Institution will accept the future drug at the offer price if the payoff from doing Nothing (the health loss from investment in R&D) is greater than the payoff to Reimbursement:

$$\overline{\Delta E^p} - \frac{f\overline{\Delta E^p}}{m} - \frac{\overline{\mathcal{R}}}{m} \geq -\frac{\overline{\mathcal{R}}}{m}$$

$$\Rightarrow \overline{\Delta E^p} - \frac{f\overline{\Delta E^p}}{m} \geq 0$$

$$\Rightarrow 1 - \frac{f}{m} \geq 0$$

$$\Rightarrow m \geq f.$$

The Institution will accept the future drug at the offer price f if there is a net increase or no net change in the population's health as a consequence of its reimbursement. Hence, at an offer price at or below m, the Institution will accept the future drug with an IPER of f.

At Stage 5 (Lobby), the Institution has a sunk cost, which can be expressed in terms of health effects:

$$\frac{\overline{\mathcal{R}}}{m}.$$

Regardless of whether the Institution chooses to Reimburse the future drug or do Nothing, it will make a loss. The Institution's objective at this stage is to minimise the loss.[8] How do we know the Institution will have a "sunk cost" in Stage 5 of the Lobby arm? In simple terms, it is the only way that the Game could have reached this point. If the Institution had not lent the funds it would not have reached this stage.[9]

---

[8] This situation analogous to impact of sunk R&D costs on the firm's decision to manufacture a new drug. Vernon et al noted that the sunk costs of R&D are "irrelevant from a firm's decision-making perspective." By the time a drug gets to market (Vernon et al. 2006).

[9] This is a critical issue in the understanding of backward induction as a solution method. See Watson (2002).

9.6.1.2 Stage 4 (Lobby): The decision to Price the New Drug

When

$$f = m,$$

the Firm maximises its profit. At this price the units of additional health effect sold
are:

$$\overline{\Delta E^p}.$$

Above this price there will be no sales, but below this price there will be no
increase in sales and hence revenue and economic profit will fall.

9.6.1.3 Stage 3 (Lobby): The Chance Node—Success or Failure of R&D

The chance node influences the expected payoff of the R&D process. For the
Institution, the expected (**E**) payoff to the Firm's decision to invest in R&D is:

$$\mathbf{E}[\Delta E] = q\left(\overline{\Delta E^p} - \frac{f\overline{\Delta E^p}}{m} - \frac{\overline{\mathcal{R}}}{m}\right) + (1-q)\left(-\frac{\overline{\mathcal{R}}}{m}\right) \tag{9.1}$$

where q is the chance outcome of R&D.

The expected effect on the population's health includes the sunk costs of
responding to Lobbying, regardless of whether R&D is successful; however, if it
is successful the Institution will also have the net benefit or the health gains for
target patients less the health effects foregone from displacing programmes to
finance the future drug.

From Stage 4 we have the result that:

$$f = m.$$

Substituting this result into Eq. (9.1), it follows that:

$$\left(\overline{\Delta E^p} - \overline{\Delta E^p} - \frac{\overline{\mathcal{R}}}{m}\right) + (1-q)\left(-\frac{\overline{\mathcal{R}}}{m}\right)$$

$$= -q\left(\frac{\overline{\mathcal{R}}}{m}\right) - \frac{\overline{\mathcal{R}}}{m} + q\left(\frac{\overline{\mathcal{R}}}{m}\right) \tag{9.2}$$

$$\Rightarrow \mathbf{E}[\Delta E] = -\frac{\overline{\mathcal{R}}}{m}.$$

That is, the Institution's expected payoff to the Firm's R&D is the loss of the sunk costs of R&D financed by the Institution.

For the Firm, the expected payoff of R&D, at an IPER $= f = m$ is:

$$\mathbf{E}[\pi_F] = q\left(m\overline{\Delta E^p} - c\overline{\Delta E^p}\right) + (1-q)(0)$$

$$= q\overline{\Delta E^p}(m-c) + 0 \qquad (9.3)$$

$$\Rightarrow \mathbf{E}[\pi_F] = q\overline{\Delta E^p}(m-c)$$

The Firm's expected economic rent (payoff) from R&D is the expected economic rent $(m\text{-}c)$ on each unit sold weighted by the probability of the successful R&D (q).

9.6.1.4 Stage 2 (Lobby): The Institution Decides Whether to Accept or Reject the Firm's Lobbying

The Institution will Accept the Lobbying if expected payoff to this action is greater than or equal to the payoff of the action N—do Nothing (reject). From Eq. (9.2), we have the expected payoff to accepting Lobby, therefore the relevant decision rule is to Accept Lobbying if:

$$-\frac{\overline{\mathcal{R}}}{m} > 0.$$

However:

$$m, \overline{\mathcal{R}} > 0$$

$$\Rightarrow -\frac{\overline{\mathcal{R}}}{m} < 0 \; \forall \; \overline{\mathcal{R}}, m.$$

Therefore there is no situation where the Institution will Accept the Lobbying.

9.6.1.5 Stage 1 (Lobby): The Firm's Payoff to Lobby

The Firm's payoff to Lobby is zero because from Stage 2 (Lobby), we see that there is no incentive for the Institution to respond to Lobbying by increasing prices.

9.6.2   Borrow

Now we consider the payoffs to the action Borrow. We start at the end of the Game at Stage 6.

9.6.2.1   Stage 6 (Borrow): The Institution's Decision to Accept the Offer Price

The situation is as for Stage 5 (Lobby) and the condition that needs to be met for the Institution to accept the future drug at the offer price is:

$$f \leq m,$$

where m is the least cost-effective in contraction of existing programmes, which, because the budget is fixed and efficient, and displacement is optimal, is the quantitative value of the health shadow price.

9.6.2.2   Stage 5 (Borrow): The Firm's Decision to Price the New Drug

The situation is as for Stage 4(Lobby) and the offer price selected by the Firm is:

$$f = m.$$

9.6.2.3   Stage 4 (Borrow): The Chance Node—Success or Failure of R&D

The expected payoff to R&D depends upon whether the Institution will reimburse the new drug. For simplification, we assume that it is profitable for the Firm to produce the drug at an IPER of m, that is, $m \geq c$. This simplification will not change the result of the Game. It is a reasonable assumption because all information is in the public domain and therefore all players know the values of m and c. Therefore, because firms will consider the price of the future drug when they make the decision to invest in R&D, they will only make this decision to invest if they expect the new drug to be profitable to manufacture.[10]

---

[10] For example Vernon et al. (2006) See footnote 7.

The expected payoff to each player is as follows:
For the Firm the expected payoff of R&D is:

$$\mathbf{E}[\pi_F] = q\left(f\overline{\Delta E^p} - c\overline{\Delta E^p} - \overline{\mathcal{R}}(1+\theta)\right) + (1-q)(0)$$
$$= q\left(f\overline{\Delta E^p} - c\overline{\Delta E^p} - \overline{\mathcal{R}}(1+\theta)\right),$$

where $f = m$, therefore the expected payoff to the Firm is:

$$\mathbf{E}[\pi_F] = q\left(\overline{\Delta E^p}(m-c) - \overline{\mathcal{R}}(1+\theta)\right). \tag{9.4}$$

This result indicates that the expected profit for the Firm is economic rent on each unit sold, less the interest and capital payment to the Capital Market and adjusted by the probability of the R&D being successful.

For the Institution the expected payoff of R&D is:

$$\mathbf{E}[\Delta E] = q\left(\overline{\Delta E^p} - \frac{f\overline{\Delta E^p}}{m}\right) + (1-q)(0),$$

where $f = m$, therefore the expected payoff is

$$\mathbf{E}[\Delta E] = q\left(\overline{\Delta E^p} - \overline{\Delta E^p}\right)$$
$$\mathbf{E}[\Delta E] = 0 \tag{9.5}$$

The payoff to the Institution is zero, regardless of the outcome of R&D, because of the profit-maximising IPER of the future drug, m, which exactly offsets the health gains foregone by displacing the least cost-effective of existing programmes.

For the Capital Market from Fig. 9.1 we see that the expected payoff of the Firm's R&D is:

$$\mathbf{E}[\pi_c] = q(\theta - \tau)\overline{\mathcal{R}} - (1-q)\overline{\mathcal{R}}(1+\tau)$$
$$= \overline{\mathcal{R}}(q\theta - q\tau - (1-q)(1+\tau))$$
$$= \overline{\mathcal{R}}(q\theta - 1 + q - \tau),$$

which can be simplified to:

$$\mathbf{E}[\pi_c] = \overline{\mathcal{R}}(q(\theta+1) - (1+\tau)). \tag{9.6}$$

The expected payoff to the Capital Market is a function of the probability of success of R&D. It is the return on the loan $\mathcal{R}$ to the Firm, at a rate θ, weighted by the probability of the success of R&D, q, less the foregone benefit of the Capital Market's zero risk alternative, which would have guaranteed a return on capital plus interest at a rate of τ. In Eq. (9.6), the expected profit is expressed as an economic rent quantum (the amount required for R&D) loaned to the Firm.

9.6.2.4 Stage 3 (Borrow): The Firm Accepts or Rejects the Capital Market's Offer of i

The Firm will accept the Capital Market's offer of θ if the Firm's expected payoff to R&D [Eq. (9.4)] is greater than or equal to zero.

$$q\left(\overline{\Delta E^p}(f - c) - \overline{\mathcal{R}}(1 + \theta)\right) \geq 0$$

where $q > 0$, therefore:

$$\overline{\Delta E^p}(f - c) - \overline{\mathcal{R}}(1 + \theta) \geq 0$$

$$\overline{\Delta E^p}(f - c) \geq \overline{\mathcal{R}}(1 + \theta) \tag{9.7}$$

$$\frac{\overline{\Delta E^p}(f - c)}{\overline{\mathcal{R}}} - 1 \geq \theta.$$

9.6.2.5 Stage 2 (Borrow): Capital Market Selects Its Offer of θ

The risk-neutral Bank will select a minimum θ, such that the expected return on the decision to lend [Eq. (9.6)] is equal to zero.[11]

$$\mathbf{E}[\pi_c] = \overline{\mathcal{R}}(q(\theta + 1) - (1 + \tau)) = 0,$$

where $\overline{\mathcal{R}} > 0$, therefore

$$q(\theta + 1) - (1 + \tau) = 0$$
$$q\theta + q - 1 - \tau = 0$$
$$q\theta = 1 - q + \tau \tag{9.8}$$
$$\theta_{min\ bank} = \frac{1 + \tau}{q} - 1.$$

The maximum acceptable θ to the Firm will occur when the Firm's expected payoff to accepting the Capital Market's price is greater than or equal to zero.

From Eq. (9.7) we have the condition:

---

[11] This is an equality because the Bank is risk neutral. See the consumer equivalent in Jehle and Reny (2001) p. 105.

$$\frac{\overline{\Delta E^p}(f-c)}{\overline{\mathcal{R}}} - 1 \geq \theta.$$

This condition provides the following maximum price:

$$\frac{\overline{\Delta E^p}(f-c)}{\overline{\mathcal{R}}} - 1 = \theta_{max\ firm}. \tag{9.9}$$

There are two possible situations for the price θ. First, if the minimum price acceptable to the Bank is more than the maximum price acceptable to the firm, the Bank could still offer its minimum acceptable price, but the loan would be refused by the Firm. This situation is described algebraically as:

$$\theta_{min\ bank} > \theta_{max\ firm}$$

We substitute in the above with Eq. (9.8) and Eq. (9.9):

$$\Rightarrow \frac{1+\tau}{q} - 1 > \frac{\overline{\Delta E^p}(f-c)}{\overline{\mathcal{R}}} - 1$$

$$\Rightarrow \frac{1+\tau}{q} > \frac{\overline{\Delta E^p}(f-c)}{\overline{\mathcal{R}}} \tag{9.10}$$

$$\Rightarrow \overline{\mathcal{R}}(1+\tau) > q\left(\overline{\Delta E^p}(f-c)\right)$$

This condition is saying that the return that the Bank could receive on a zero-risk loan of $\overline{\mathcal{R}}$:

$$\overline{\mathcal{R}}(1+\tau)$$

is more than the expected additional rent

$$q\left(\overline{\Delta E^p}(f-c)\right)$$

that the Firm can make on its investment of $\overline{\mathcal{R}}$. In this case we assume that the Capital Market makes an offer to the Firm of:

$$\theta_{min\ bank} = \frac{1+\tau}{q} - 1,$$

which the Firm will not accept.

The second possible situation is if the minimum price acceptable by the Bank is less than the maximum price acceptable to the Firm, in which case the resultant equilibrium price θ^* will be between these two and will depend upon the relative bargaining powers of the Firm and the Bank.

That is:

$$\theta_{min\ bank} \leq \theta^* \leq \theta_{max\ firm}.$$

9.6.2.6   Stage 1 Should the Firm Borrow, Lobby or Do Nothing?

The key strategic decision is whether the Firm should Lobby, Borrow or do Nothing. To establish the conditions under which the Firm will select from these three options, the payoffs to each are calculated. What will determine this choice?

> **Note** The pharma-economic literature recognises the influence of future price on a firm's decision to invest in R&D. For example Vernon et al. point out that if firms had not expected prices that would cover R&D they would not have made this investment (Vernon et al. 2006, p. 182). This dynamic GTM also recognises this issue. This Game also recognises that the Institution will take into consideration future prices in their payoff to accepting lobbying today. The latter analogous fact is not widely, if at all, recognised in the pharma-economic literature.

Payoff to Do Nothing

The payoff from the Game for all players from the Firm choosing to do Nothing is zero.

Payoff to Lobby

The expected payoff to the Firm of Lobby is zero. There is no incentive for the Institution to invest in R&D via a higher price today. The reason is that there is no mechanism whereby the Institution can recoup its initial investment in R&D via higher prices for the existing drug.

Payoff to Borrow

If the minimum acceptable interest rate for the Bank is higher than the maximum acceptable rate for the Firm, then there will be no payoff to Borrow. These conditions are presented in Eq. (9.10).In this case the Firm will chose to do Nothing. However, if this condition is not met, then the Firm will choose to Borrow and the expected payoff will be:

$$E[\pi_F] = q\left(\overline{\Delta E^P}(f - c) - \overline{\mathcal{R}}(1 + \theta^*)\right) \tag{9.11}$$

where we assume:

$$\theta_{min\ bank} \leq \theta^* \leq \theta_{max\ firm}.$$

Substituting Eq. (9.8) and Eq. (9.9) we have:

$$\frac{1+\tau}{q} \leq \theta^* \leq \frac{\overline{\Delta E^P}(f - c)}{\overline{\mathcal{R}} - 1}$$

Therefore the expected payoff per unit sold to the Firm from Borrow (given that it is greater than zero) is between the profit at the maximum interest rate and the profit at the minimum interest rate, where the profit for the Firm as a function of θ is sourced from Eq. (9.4).

$$q\left(\overline{\Delta E^P}(f - c) - \overline{\mathcal{R}}\left(\frac{1 + \overline{\Delta E^P}(f - c)}{\overline{\mathcal{R}}} - 1\right)\right) \leq E[\pi_F] \leq q\left(\overline{\Delta E^P}(f - c) - \overline{\mathcal{R}}\left(1 + \frac{1 + \tau}{q}\right)\right)$$

$$\Rightarrow 0 \leq E[\pi_F] \leq q\left(\overline{\Delta E^P}(f - c) - \overline{\mathcal{R}}\left(1 + \frac{1 + \tau}{q}\right)\right)$$

$$\Rightarrow 0 \leq E[\pi_F] \leq q\overline{\Delta E^P}(f - c) - \overline{\mathcal{R}}(q + 1 + \tau).$$

That is, the expected payoff to the Firm is between zero (if the Bank appropriates the entire surplus and charges at the Firm's maximum θ) and the additional profit $(f\text{-}c)$ from each unit of health effects sold $\overline{\Delta E^P}$, adjusted by the probability of Success of R&D (q) less the costs of borrowing R&D funding at the Bank's minimum θ.

9.6.3 Equilibrium

What are the conditions at equilibrium? The equilibrium result will depend upon whether there is an interest rate that provides an incentive for the Firm to Borrow and the Bank to lend. If there is no such rate, then the equilibrium result is no action and the payoff is zero for all players. However if there is an incentive for the Firm to Borrow and the Bank to lend, then there will be a payoff greater than zero to the Firm and/or Capital Market.

The expected payoff to the Firm will be a function of θ:

$$0 \leq \mathbf{E}[\pi_F] \leq q\overline{\Delta E^p}(f - c) - \overline{\mathcal{R}}(q + 1 + \tau).$$

The expected payoff to the Capital Market is also a function of θ:

$$\mathbf{E}[\pi_C] = \theta\overline{\mathcal{R}}$$

$$\mathbf{E}[\pi_C] = \overline{\mathcal{R}}\left(\frac{1}{q} - 1\right).$$

And the expected payoff to the Institution will be:

$$\mathbf{E}[\Delta E] = \overline{\Delta E^p} - \frac{f\overline{\Delta E^p}}{m},$$

where:

$$f = m$$

$$\therefore \mathbf{E}[\Delta E] = \overline{\Delta E^p} - \overline{\Delta E^p} = 0.$$

So at equilibrium, regardless of whether the Firm chooses Borrow or No Action, there is no net increase in the health of the population. This outcome is a consequence of the Firm's incentive to price at the threshold IPER and the Institution's lack of capacity to bargain below this price. In conclusion, EVCI from the development of the new drug, if it exists, will be shared between the Capital Market and the Firm.

9.7   Discussion

Firms claim the reason that they rely on economic rent to source their R&D funds is because banks are unwilling to lend at a rate that allows firms to be profitable. This state of the world is consistent with the situation described in the Game where the minimum interest rate required by the Bank is higher than the maximum interest rate that the Firm can pay and still be profitable. This Game shows that if this situation exists there is no incentive for the Institution to increase prices to finance this R&D because there are no mechanisms whereby this investment by the institution can be recouped.

But there is one more option suggested by this Game; the Firm could offer to contract with the Institution, which can recoup its initial investment $\mathcal{R}$. This contract could be in the form of a discount on the IPER of the future drug, which would otherwise be β_c, which in this case has a quantitative value of m. The Game can be used to predict whether the Institution will be willing to enter such a contract by taking into account the risk preferences of the Institution relative to those of the Capital Market. If the Institution appropriately accommodated the risks (as the Capital Market does) and had the same attitude to risk as the Capital Market, then it is unclear why we would expect the payoff to the Firm to contracting with the Institution to be higher than the payoff to the strategy Borrow. The reason for this lack of clarity is that the Institution would require the same minimum share of surplus should the R&D be successful as the Capital Market requires, in addition to recouping its initial investment. Under this situation, the cost advantages to the Firm of the strategy Lobby relative to the strategy "Borrow" would be removed.

This conclusion—the Institution requires at least the same benefit as the Capital Market to have an incentive to invest—appears counterintuitive; the Institution can benefit from the additional future health effects whereas the Capital Market does not. It is true that if the Institution were provided with the additional health effects at no net financial cost ($\Delta C^P < 0$) then there would be an additional incentive for the Institution. However, the Institution is required to pay for these additional health gains (possibly at or above β_c) as well as finance the R&D. At β_c the Institution is indifferent between health effects from the new drug and health effects purchased through other strategies. Therefore, there is only one way the Institution can be made better off by contracting compared with relying on the Firm to Borrow from the Capital Market. This incentive is: a return on their investment $\mathcal{R}$ (via a lower future price) and an additional incentive of a further discount on the price to account for the risk.

If institutions, the agent of consumers, are more risk-averse than the Capital Market, then we would expect that institutions would require a higher value of θ to accommodate the risks of R&D, compared with that required by the Capital Market. Hence, the Firm's return on Borrow could be higher than the return on Lobby and Contract with the Institution.

In conclusion, if EVCI > 0, then by entering into a contract to be paid a share of this surplus in addition to being repaid the capital, an incentive for the Institution to provide the funds to the Firm is generated. However, it is likely that in order for the relatively risk-averse Institution[12] to be willing to enter such a contract, it will need to be compensated for undertaking the loan, and this compensation would need to be more than that required by the risk-neutral Capital Market. Hence, if risks are appropriately accommodated by the Institution, the Firm is predicted to prefer the strategy Borrow to those of Lobby and Contract.

In the real world, we observe that a Firm sources its R&D from internal funds raised by economic rent which in turn results from Lobbying. Does this mean the Game has poor predictive value? In the polite language of Game Theory, the Institution has made a "mistake" rather than acted "irrationally".[13] The observation

---

[12] More risk averse than the Bank and not a risk taker.

[13] A mistake is an error made by a player, possibly a result of the complexities of a strategy. For example see Watson (2002) p. 27. The idea of irrationality could suggest that the player is acting in

that it is cheaper to source funds internally is a consequence of a mistake by the Institution in providing these funds and not requiring a return; the failure is by the Institution not the Capital Market.

The Game reveals that if the Firm knows that there is a possibility that the Institution will make a mistake in its response to lobbying, then there is an incentive for the Firm to Lobby in order to gain the funds for R&D at a cheaper rate (no interest) plus no requirement to repay the capital. Furthermore, the evidence suggests that only some of the funds raised by lobbying are invested in NME R&D, between 20 and 30 % (Reinhardt 2007). There is a cost to lobbying. However, the returns to the Firm in excess of the funds invested in lobbying and the savings compared with the strategy of Borrow makes Lobby a very effective strategy. The ostensibly evidence-based Threat, that the population will be worse off if it does not finance R&D through higher prices, is an effective tactic within this strategy of Lobbying. Investing in the evidence to support this Threat is also an important part of the strategy of Lobbying.

And finally, if the Institution provides the funds to the Firm in a situation where there is no interest rate that was acceptable to both the Firm and the Capital Market, then there is a deadweight social loss if the Institution responds to Lobbying. Society would have been better off if these funds had instead been invested by the Institution into other strategies, for example, the development of unpatentable but very cost-effective innovation(aICER $< \beta_c$). This issue is addressed in more detail in the following chapter.

9.8   Conclusion

Drug companies and pharma-economists use a range of arguments to defend the position that institutions should not use their monopsony power to negotiate a price below the FPP. Some of these arguments are contradictory. For example, firms and pharma-economists argue that firms need to be compensated for the risky investments that they make into pharmaceutical R&D. However, at the same time firms argue that they need to finance R&D for future drugs from internal funds because the capital markets will not bear this risk. These internal funds are sourced from above marginal cost pricing of drugs. There are no contracts or agreements for firms to repay this investment by, for example, lowering the price of the future drug,

---

a way that is not consistent with their objectives. The idea of players acting rationally is significant in game theory because it is the assumption that allows players to select their own strategy based on the expected response by the other player. There could still be strategic uncertainty in the other player's response, even if all players act rationally. It is unusual in Game Theory to assume that there is only one definition of rationality, but some concepts of rationality dominate. (See Watson 2002 and Grüne-Yanoff and Schweinzer 2008) Games however can incorporate the idea of mistakes and in Evolutionary Game Theory mistakes can play a significant role in achieving an evolutionary stable equilibrium. See Samuelson (2002).

therefore the purchasers not only bear the risks of this investment, they bear the entire costs and the risks.

The Reimburser is convinced by Game 2 that the observation that firms finance their R&D from internal funds does not mean that unless firms access these internal funds through higher prices, there will be either no R&D, or less R&D, and the health of the future population will be worse. She also recognises that only 20–30 % of these additional funds finance NME R&D and therefore the benefits to the Firm of the strategy of Lobby are underestimated by focusing on the return of future profit alone.

However, the Reimburser is still reluctant to accept that there is no benefit to the population's health from adjusting β_c to take into account the relationship between price and innovation. But how should it be taken into account?

Jena and Philipson (2008) proposed that there should be a premium paid for health effects purchased from new drug manufacturers because the purchaser is buying both current technology health effects and future technologies, whereas for other services the purchaser is only buying health effects from current technologies. This strategy would effectively be a premium over β_c. In the following chapter this proposition for a decision threshold plus premium for new drugs is analysed in a dynamic three-stage game that explores the incentive for an Institution to move away from β_c as the decision threshold.

The following chapter also explores the possibility that overall social welfare (economic rent plus consumer welfare) will be higher if the Institution pays a premium, even if the population's health is worse. This methodological issue was one of the findings of the review of the pharma-economic literature presented in Pekarsky (2012, Appendix 2).

References

Cook JP, Vernon JA, Manning R (2008) Pharmaceutical risk-sharing agreements. PharmacoEconomics 26:551–556

Grüne-Yanoff T, Schweinzer P (2008) The roles of stories in applying game theory. J Econ Methodol 15(2):131–146

Hall BH (2002) The financing of research and development. Oxf Rev Econ Policy 18(1):35–51. doi:10.1093/oxrep/18.1.35

International Trade Administration (2004) Pharmaceutical price controls in OECD countries: implications for U.S. consumers, pricing, research and development, and innovation. International Trade Administration, Washington, DC

Jehle G, Reny P (2001) Advanced microeconomic theory. Addison Wesley, Boston, MA

Jena AB, Philipson TJ (2008) Cost-effectiveness analysis and innovation. J Health Econ 27:1224–1236

Pekarsky BAK (2012) Trust, constraints and the counterfactual: reframing the political economy of new drug price. Dissertation, University of Adelaide http://digital.library.adelaide.edu.au/dspace/handle/2440/79171. Accessed 25 Dec 2013

Reinhardt U (2001) Perspectives on the pharmaceutical industry. Health Aff 20(5):136–149

Reinhardt U (2007) The pharmaceutical sector in health care. In: Sloan F, Hsieh C-R (eds) Pharmaceutical innovation: incentives, competition, and cost-benefit analysis in international perspective. Cambridge University Press, New York

Samuelson L (2002) Evolution and game theory. J Econ Perspect 16(2):47–66

Santerre RE, Vernon JA (2006) Assessing consumer gains from a drug price control policy in the United States. South Econ J 73(1):233–245

Congressional Budget Office US (2006) Research and development in the pharmaceutical industry. The US Congress, Washington, DC

Vernon JA (2003) Price regulation, capital market imperfections, and strategic R&D investment behavior in the pharmaceutical industry: consequences for innovation. University of Pennsylvania, Philadelphia, PA

Vernon JA, Golec JH, Hughen WK (2006) The economics of pharmaceutical price regulation and importation: refocusing the debate. Am J Law Med 32(2–3):175–192

Watson J (2002) Strategy: an introduction to game theory. W. W. Norton and Company, New York

Chapter 10
The "Pharmacotherapy Needs a Premium" Game

Abstract This chapter presents "The pharmacotherapy needs a premium" Game where the Institution that lowers the decision threshold must respond to the industry's Threat. The pharmaceutical industry's claim is that while the health shadow price β_c captures information about the budget constraint and can improve static efficiency in a fixed budget, β_c does not capture information about the loss in future health as a consequence of lower drug prices today. The industry claims that new drugs should have a premium above the threshold for other programmes because when a fund holder buys new drugs they are also buying future innovation. The Game is structured as a Firm's choice between two strategies: (1) invest in research and development; or (2) do nothing. The Game extends over three periods and up to two drugs (a new drug and a future drug) can be developed. The key decision by the Institution is whether or not to pay a premium over β_c for the new drug (the first drug) in order to facilitate development of the future (second) drug. The result of the Game is that there is no incentive for an Institution to price above β_c for the new drug in order to generate an incentive for the Firm to develop the future drug. Furthermore, pricing above β_c is found to be neither a necessary nor sufficient condition for the development of the future drug. I conclude that the Institution should respond to the Threat by suggesting that the Firm approach the Capital Market and that this is the social-welfare-maximising solution.

10.1 The Reimburser's Problem

The Reimburser is presented with a new drug by a pharmaceutical Firm. The new drug is more effective than the best existing drug, $\Delta E^P > 0$ but it also comes at an additional financial cost, $\Delta C^P > 0$. In order to finance the new drug within the fixed economically efficient health budget, an existing programme needs to be displaced; the least cost-effective of existing programmes. However, this existing programme has an aICER less than the IPER of the new drug ($m < f$), therefore, the health effects displaced to finance the new drug will be more than the health effects gained from reimbursing the new drug. Furthermore, the budget is currently economically efficient and displacement is optimal so, using PEA, the threshold is $\beta_c = d = m$,

© Springer International Publishing Switzerland 2015
B.A.K. Pekarsky, *The New Drug Reimbursement Game*,
DOI 10.1007/978-3-319-08903-4_10

where d is the aICER of an optimally displaced service and m is the aICER of the least cost-effective in contraction of an existing programme.

The Reimburser is reluctant to choose to reimburse the new drug in this situation. However, the Firm presents the Reimburser with a paper by pharma-economists Jena and Philipson (2008) who propose that new pharmaceuticals should have a higher threshold applied to them than non-pharmaceutical inputs. The authors' reasoning is that purchasing the former is simply buying health effects from current technologies whereas purchasing new drugs has the benefits of both current health effects and future innovation. They claim that the product with the worst cost-effectiveness could also be the one that maximises health and status and dynamic efficiency. They suggest that the choice is not between "a cheap or expensive technologies once marketed—as CE adoption suggests."[1] Instead the choice is one between an "initially expensive technology and no technology" and if the latter is chosen then society is also choosing a future with "higher real prices for producing a healthy life" (Jena and Philipson 2008, p. 1235).

The Reimburser recognises that the programme that will be displaced to finance the additional costs of the new drug does not have an R&D component, so there appears to be little potential to change the efficiency of future health budgets through improved technology via this programme. Jena and Philipson's conclusion has intuitive appeal: why not pay a bit extra for a new drug, given that we are getting more than just the health effects of that drug? The Reimburser asks her Health Economic Adviser how the Institution should respond to the following Threat.

> When the Institution buys this new drug, it buys the health effects from this drug and the health benefits from future innovation. This is not the case with other health programmes. Therefore, unless the Institution pays a premium for the health effects from the new drug, the population will be worse off because innovation will be suboptimal and the future drug will not be produced.

10.2   The Pharmacotherapy Needs a Premium Game

Chapter 8 presented a one-period GTM of the reimbursement process. The following Game extends that one-period model to a three-period model where the decisions linking successive time periods are the Firm's decision to invest today in the R&D required for future drugs and the Reimburser's decision to change the threshold price in order to change the availability of future NMEs.

---

[1] It is unclear whether the authors are conflating the ideas of cheap and expensive technologies and cost-effective and cost-ineffective technologies unintentionally.

This game is set out in the following four Sects. (10.3 to 10.6). Section 10.3 describes the World from which the problem characterised by the same is drawn. In Sect. 10.4 the model is described and defined, first in terms of the Narrative then the structure of the applied game. The theory used to derive the solution is described in Sect. 10.5 and the Solution is presented in Sect. 10.6.

10.3   The World

In 2008 a Firm developed a new drug, Araamax for rheumatoid arthritis. The evidence from double-blinded RCTs showed a statistically and clinically significant gain to a subgroup of patients compared with the existing best therapy, Rathmab. Purchasing Araamax will come at a significant additional cost to the health care sector, ΔC^P, which will be financed by displacing an existing programme. The aICER of the displaced programme is less than the IPER of the new drug so there will be a net loss in the population's health. However, the Firm claims that because the new drug has both dynamic and static welfare implications whereas the existing programme has only the latter, the new drug should be purchased at the offer price despite the short-term reduction in the health effects for the population.[2]

The Firm makes the following Threat.

> When the Institution buys this new drug, it buys the health effects from this drug and the health benefits from future innovation. This is not the case with other health programmes. Therefore, unless the Institution pays a premium for the health effects from the new drug, the population will be worse off because innovation will be suboptimal and the future drug will not be produced.

How should the Institution respond to this Threat?

10.4   The Model

The Model comprises the Narrative and the Game Structure.

---

[2] By static efficiency the authors are referring to the aICER of the current budget and current technologies. The capacity for innovation to change dynamic efficiency refers to its influence on the aICER of a future budget.

10.4.1   The Narrative

The Game takes place over three periods. Currently patients with rheumatoid arthritis use a drug called Rathmab which is off-patent and hence its IPER, compared with placebo, is the same as its IMER; there is no economic rent. It is produced by a different firm from the one in this Game.

> **Note**
> The relationship between the IMER, IPER and IπER of each of the three drugs is illustrated using numeric values for variables in Tables 10.1, 10.2, 10.3, 10.4 and 10.5. The Game is solved algebraically and hence these values are illustrative only. These numbers are referenced in brackets and italics throughout the narrative.

10.4.1.1   Period 1

The Game starts in Period 1 when the Firm makes a decision about whether to invest a fixed research budget financed by internal funds into pharmaceutical R&D or do nothing. The Firm's objective is to maximise economic rent. If the Firm invests in R&D, at the end of Period 1 they will have a new drug (Araamax) for

Table 10.1 Clinical innovation per course measured in QALYs for three drugs compared to their up to three alternatives: a hypothetical example

Comparison	Rathmab (R)	Araamax (A)	Araamaxplus (A+)
Compared to placebo (QALYs)	$0.05_{(d)}$	$0.1_{(d)}$	0.22
Compared to Rathmab (QALYs)	n/a	$0.05_{(e)}$	0.17
Compared to Araamax (QALYs)	n/a	n/a	0.12

This table indicates the clinical innovation of the drug named in the column with that of each less effective option labelled in the rows. The subscript letters in brackets (e.g. (d)) refer to the text in this section. Each successive drug is clinically innovative compared to placebo and the previous best available drug and also contains the clinical innovation of the previous drug(s). (d) and (e) refer to the text following these tables in Sects. 10.4.1.2 and 10.4.1.5.

Table 10.2 Price, manufacturing cost and economic rent per course for three: a hypothetical example

	Rathmab (R)	Araamax (A)	Araamaxplus (A+)
Price per course ($)	250	4,000	13,000
Cost of manufacture per course ($)	$250_{(c)}$	$500_{(c)}$	$620_{(h)}$
Economic rent per course ($)	0	3,500	12,380

The price per course is derived from the IPER. In this case the price of A and A + is based on an IPER of $75,000 per QALY. The cost of manufacturing a course of the drug increases for each successive drug due to changes in the methods of manufacturing. It includes a normal profit. The economic rent on each course sold is simply the revenue from sales less the cost of manufacturing course of the drug. (c) and (h) refer to the text following these tables in Sects. 10.4.1.2 and 10.4.1.5.

Table 10.3 Incremental price per incremental health effect (IPER) for three drugs against different comparators: a hypothetical example

Comparison	Rathmab (R)	Araamax (A)	Araamaxplus (A+)
Compared to placebo ($)	5,000	40,000	59,091
Compared to Rathmab ($)	n/a	75,000(a)	75,000
Compared to Araamax ($)	n/a	n/a	75,000

The IPER for R is the same as the cost of manufacturing because the drug is off patent. The IPER for clinical innovation of both A and A + is $75,000. A + is paid an IPER of $75,000 for both its own innovative QALYs and those of A. *(a)* refers to the text following these tables in Sects. 10.4.1.2 and 10.4.1.5.

Table 10.4 Incremental manufacturing cost per additional QALY for three drugs against different comparators: a hypothetical example

Comparison	Rathmab (R)	Araamax (A)	Araamaxplus (A+)
Compared to placebo ($)	5,000(b)	5,000(f)	2,818(k)
Compared to Rathmab ($)	n/a	5,000(j)	2,176(n)
Compared to Araamax ($)	n/a	n/a	1,000(i)

The IMER of R is the cost of manufacturing per QALY compared to placebo. Both A and A + are clinically innovative, however, in this example, only A + has innovation in manufacturing also; the IMER of A + versus A is only $1,000 compared to the IMER of $5,000 of the previous two drugs. *(b)*, *(f)*, *(j)*, *(k)* and *(n)* refers to the text following these tables in Sects. 10.4.1.2 and 10.4.1.5.

Table 10.5 Incremental economic rent per additional QALY for three drugs against different comparators: a hypothetical example

Comparison	Rathmab (R) ($)	Araamax (A) ($)	Araamaxplus (A+) ($)
Compared to placebo	–	35,000(l)	56,273(m)
Compared to Rathmab	n/a	70,000(g)	72,824
Compared to Araamax	n/a	n/a	74,000

The IπER of R is zero because the drug is off patent. Significantly, because A is on patent when it A + is reimbursed, A is able to capture the economic rent on the clinical innovation of both A and A+. *(g)*, *(l)*, and *(m)* refers to the text following these tables in Sects. 10.4.1.2 and 10.4.1.5.

rheumatoid arthritis. This new drug will have an additional clinical benefit compared with the best existing pharmaco-therapy (Rathmab). This additional effect is for a sub-group of patients and is a reduction in pain and stiffness to a threshold that allows normal daily living. The additional effect is experienced by: (1) all patients in the sub-group who receive the drug (intervention); (2) no patients in the sub-group who do not receive the drug (the control group); and (3) no patients who receive this drug but are outside this sub-group (control and intervention).

10.4.1.2   Period 2

If the Firm does invest in R&D in Period 1, then at the start of the Period 2, the Firm offers the Institution the new drug, Araamax, which has an IPER calculated relative to the best existing drug, Rathmab *($75,000(a)* Table 10.3). Rathmab is currently priced at its IMER (which his equivalent to pricing at marginal cost); calculated relative to placebo. ($5,000$_{(b)}$ Table 10.4) The cost of producing a vial of Araamax is more than the cost of producing a vial of Rathmab. ($500 > 250_{(c)}$ Table 10.2) Each vial of Araamax "contains" more health effects compared with placebo than a vial of Rathmab compared with placebo. ($0.1 > 0.05$_{(d)}$ Table 10.1) This is the clinical innovation of Araamax. ($0.1 - 0.05 = 0.05$_{(e)}$ Table 10.1) Therefore the IMER of Araamax (compared with Rathmab)[3] is greater than zero ($250/0.05 = $5,000 > 0$_{(f)}$ Table 10.4) and is assumed to be the same as the IMER for Rathmab (compared with placebo) ($5,000$_{(b)}$ Table 10.4). This means there is clinical innovation (more health effects per vial) but no manufacturing innovation (the incremental costs of manufacturing each incremental health gain is the same for Araamax versus Rathmab and Rathmab versus placebo).

The Firm makes no economic rent on the non-clinically innovative units of Araamax because these are priced at their IMER. However, on every unit of additional health effect (Araamax compared with Rathmab) sold, the difference in the IPER and the IMER of these additional health effects represents economic rent to the Firm on the innovative health effects, the IπER ($75,000 - $5,000 = $70,000$_{(g)}$ Table 10.5).

The Institution can choose to reimburse Araamax or do nothing. The Institution seeks to maximise the health of the population given the existing budget. If the Institution is indifferent to the payoff of reimbursement compared with that for doing nothing, it must choose to reimburse. If the Institution chooses to reimburse Araamax, it will reimburse it for all patients who are in the sub-group for which there is an effect. None of the patients who currently have their access to Rathmab subsidised will continue to be prescribed Rathmab. Instead they will all be pre-scribed Araamax, which is clinically superior. If Araamax is not reimbursed, no patients will have the new drug due to its very high annual cost (around 75 % of the average salary of a person with severe RA).[4] In this way the health effect of the policy to reimburse Araamax is discrete rather than continuous.

The Institution, which has a fixed budget, must displace existing services to finance the additional cost of the new drug for every year that Araamax continues to be the best available pharmaco-therapy for these patients. Furthermore, once Araamax is reimbursed, it cannot be displaced until a new drug that is clinically superior for this group of patients is reimbursed; Araamax cannot be displaced to finance a different programme or a new drug for which it is not a clinical substitute. The health budget is allocatively efficient at the start of Period 2; there is no alternative allocation of resources across existing inputs and technologies that can improve health outcomes for the population. There is also no investment in

---

[3] The IMER of Araamax relative to Rathmab the additional cost of manufacturing the additional health effects in each vial.

[4] In 2005, the cost of etanercept (a disease modifying agent) was estimated at £178.75 per dose, 52 doses of 50 mg per year, which is £9,295 per year (Chen et al. 2006). A person with severe RA is likely to earn less than the average salary, therefore it is conceivable that a new RA drug could be more than 75 % of the salary of a person with severe RA.

improved practice that can be made today that will have returns of a lower aICER for a programme in the future that offsets the health effects foregone today due to the initial investment. Finally, if Araamax is reimbursed, it is financed by optimal displacement ($d = m$). The contracted programme is unpatented and continuous, that is, it can be contracted or expanded by any unit and there will be a corresponding decrease or increase in health effects.

If Araamax is reimbursed at the start of Period 2 then the Firm will produce it at an IMERc_1 ($\$5,000_{(f)}$ Table 10.4). At the start of Period 2 the Firm has to decide whether it will use some of the economic rent from the production and sale of Araamax to develop a new RA drug, or whether it will no longer innovate and simply continue to produce Araamax. The Firm's payoff to continuing to manufacture Araamax will be the economic rent from the sale of the drug in Periods 2 and 3. If the Firm decides to invest in the development of a new RA drug, it will incur a cost of R&D in Period 2 in addition to the cost of manufacturing Araamax. It will also be in receipt of the revenue from the sales of Araamax in Period 2.

10.4.1.3   Period 3

If the Firm chose not to invest in R&D in Period 2 then in Period 3 the Firm continues to manufacture Araamax and the Institution continues to displace services to finance its additional cost and reimburse Araamax for eligible patients.

If the Firm chose to invest in R&D in Period 2 then at the end of Period 2 the Firm has a new drug, Araamaxplus, a more effective drug than Araamax. The gain compared with Araamax is both clinically and statistically significant. It works for the same patient group as for Araamax and if Araamaxplus is approved for reimbursement then all patients who currently receive Araamax will instead be prescribed Araamaxplus. If the Institution chooses to reimburse Araamaxplus it must displace additional services to finance the additional cost of these additional health effects.

10.4.1.4   Political Economy

This narrative contains two aspects of the political economy of the reimbursement process.

1. If the Institution is indifferent between reimbursing the new drug and continuing funding the existing drug, it must select the new drug.
2. The Institution cannot displace a drug that it has reimbursed to finance care for the same or different group of patients; it can only replace it with a superior drug for the same patient group.

10.4.1.5   The Relationship Between IMERs, IPERs, Expenditure and Costs of Manufacturing

This Game introduces the possibility that a future drug can have both clinical and manufacturing innovation; a reduction in the average cost of manufacturing each incremental QALY compared to either placebo or the previous drug. It also demonstrates how successive drugs capture the economic rent of previous drugs as a consequence of the combined effect of new drugs being introduced before comparators are off-patent and the application of CEA_i.

Tables 10.1 to 10.5 set out a hypothetical example of the drugs that this Game characterises. These tables illustrate some of the characteristics of IMER, IPERs and IπERs in the case of drugs reimbursed successively. Araamaxplus has clinical innovation. If Araamax is still on patent and the IPER > IMER[5] then the economic rent appropriated by the Firm in relation to the clinically innovative health effects of Araamax relative to Rathmab ($\$70,000_{(g)}$ Table 10.5), are also available on the sale of Araamaxplus. This is in addition to the IπER available on the clinically innovative health effects of Araamaxplus compared with Araamax. (See Pekarsky [2012, Appendix 6) for a discussion of the appropriation of first drug in class surplus by subsequent drugs.]

Now consider the consequences for the IπER of Araamaxplus (compared to Araamax) if there is manufacturing innovation. The additional cost of manufacturing a course of Araamax relative to Rathmab ($\$500_{(c)} - \$250_{(c)} = \$250$ Table 10.2) is more than the additional cost of manufacturing a course of Araamaxplus relative to Araamax ($\$620_{(h)} - \$500_{(c)} = \$120$ Table 10.2). Also, Araamaxplus has an IMER on the innovative units relative to Araamax ($\$1,000_{(i)}$ Table 10.4) that is less than the IMER of the clinically innovative units of Araamax relative to Rathmab ($\$5,000_{(f)}$ Table 10.4). Therefore there is manufacturing innovation relative to both Rathmab ($\$2,818_{(k)} < \$5,000_{(b)}$ Table 10.4) and Araamax ($\$2,176_{(n)} < \$5,000_{(f)}$ Table 10.4). This innovation reduces the average cost of producing additional health effects. The IPER is the same for the innovative units of Araamax and Araamaxplus, Araamaxplus appropriates Araamax's economic rent and the average cost of manufacture of all of these health effects is reduced. Hence, the economic rent on all clinically innovative health effects relative to placebo is increased for Araamaxplus compared with Araamax ($\$35,000_{(l)} < \$56,273_{(m)}$ Table 10.5). This means that with the same conventionally calculated IPER for Araamaxplus and Araamax, the economic rent for the new drug is higher due to the effect of the manufacturing innovation.

---

[5] The IMER = IPER if there is perfect competition in the generic drug market and the drug is off-patent. If the drug is on patent, the IPER could still be equal to the IMER. This situation is a consequence of the choice of threshold IPER and the cost function for the drug, which can be assumed to be independent. However, provided that the Firm only produces and sells the drug if it makes a normal profit, then the IMER cannot be greater than the IPER.

10.4.2 Game Structure

There are two players (the Firm and the Institution). It is a dynamic (consecutive decisions) three-period game of complete (public) and perfect (no uncertainty) information, therefore both players know the value of all parameters and variables with certainty at the start of the game. (We will relax these assumptions in the discussion). The game is represented as an extensive form game in Fig. 10.1.

10.4.2.1 Strategies and Payoffs

The Game starts with the Firm.

Firm

The Firm has five possible actions: Develop a new drug (D); Develop a new drug and manufacture the current drug (D&M); price the new or future drug f; manufacture the new drug only (M); or do nothing (N).

At the start of Period 1, the Firm can choose to Develop (D) or do Nothing (N). If it chooses to Develop, at the end of Period 1 it can then choose a price f_1 for the first new drug, Araamax. If the Institution chooses to reimburse the new drug at the offer price, at the start of Period 2 the Firm can then choose to either develop a second drug, Araamaxplus, while continuing to manufacture and sell Araamax (D&M) or manufacture Araamax only (M). If it develops Araamaxplus (the future drug), it must choose a price f_2 for Araamaxplus when it goes to the market at the end of Period 2.

The pay-off to the Firm from N is zero. If the Firm chooses to develop Araamax but it is not reimbursed by the Institution, its payoff is a loss of $\overline{\mathcal{R}}$, the fixed cost of developing a new drug. The Firm's payoff if it manufactures and sells Araamax for two periods and does not develop a second drug is the sum of the economic rent over Periods 2 and 3:

$$\pi_2 + \pi_3 = 2f_1\overline{\Delta E} - 2c_1\overline{\Delta E} - \overline{\mathcal{R}} \tag{10.1}$$

where the revenue $2c_1\overline{\Delta E}_1$ comprises the sales of health gains $\overline{\Delta E}_1$ at price f_1 over these two periods less the fixed cost of R&D $\overline{\mathcal{R}}$ and the variable cost of manufacturing $c_1\overline{\Delta E}_1$.

Finally, the economic rent in Periods 1 to 3 if Araamaxplus is developed in Period 2 and is reimbursed by the Institution is:

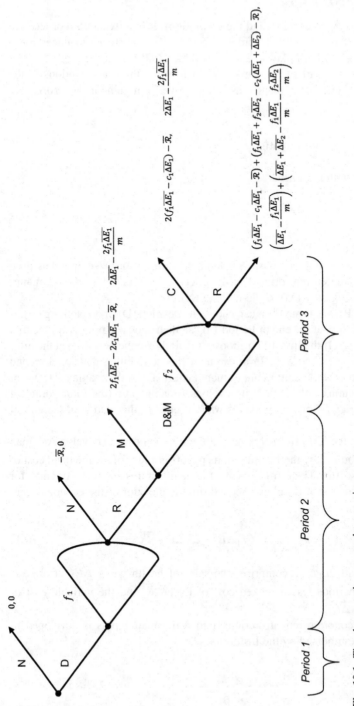

Fig. 10.1 The pharmacotherapy needs a premium game

$$\pi_2 + \pi_3 = \left(f_1 \overline{\Delta E}_1 - c_1 \overline{\Delta E}_1 - \overline{\mathcal{R}} \right)$$
$$+ \left(f_1 \overline{\Delta E}_1 + f_2 \overline{\Delta E}_2 - c_2 \left(\overline{\Delta E}_1 + \overline{\Delta E}_2 \right) - \overline{\mathcal{R}} \right) \qquad (10.2)$$

where:

- Araamaxplus has gains of $\overline{\Delta E}_1 + \overline{\Delta E}_2$ compared with the original drug Rathmab, and $\overline{\Delta E}_2$ compared with Araamax.
- The health effects $\overline{\Delta E}_1$ of Araamaxplus (which are appropriated from Araamax) are sold at the IPER that was used for Araamax (f_1) whereas the IPER of $\overline{\Delta E}_2$ (the health gain of Araamaxplus compared with Araamax) is f_2. This situation is a consequence of the sequential reimbursement decisions that are always based on the IPER of the new drug versus the existing drug. (See Table 10.5 and Pekarsky (2012, Appendix 6)). Therefore the revenue in Period 3 from the sales of Araamaxplus is:

$$f_1 \overline{\Delta E}_1 + f_2 \overline{\Delta E}_2$$

- Producing the additional health effects compared with Rathmab $\left(\overline{\Delta E}_1 + \overline{\Delta E}_2 \right)$ has a cost of c_2 per unit of health effect. Therefore c_2 is the IMER of Araamaxplus compared with Rathmab.
- Therefore the economic rent on the sales of Araamaxplus is the revenue per unit (the IPER) less the variable cost of manufacture of each additional unit (the IMER) multiplied by the number of units of effect less the fixed cost of R&D ($\overline{\mathcal{R}}$).

10.4.2.2   Institution

The Institution has three possible actions: do Nothing (N) in relation to the offer price for Araamax or Araamaxplus, Reimburse (R) the new drug being offered by the Firm at the offer price or Continue (C), continue to reimburse Araamax in Period 3 rather than Reimburse Araamaxplus.

The Institution's payoff to do Nothing when offered Araamax at the end of Period 1 is zero.

The Institution's payoff to the action of Reimburse, R, then Continue, C, (Reimbursing Araamax at the offer price and continuing to purchase it over the next two periods with no offer of a second drug) is the net increase in the population's health:

$$\Delta E = 2 \overline{\Delta E}_1 - \frac{2 f_1 \overline{\Delta E}_1}{m},$$

where $2 \overline{\Delta E}_1$ is the health effects of Araamax compared with Rathmab over two periods, for the target patients and:

$$\frac{2f_1\overline{\Delta E}_1}{m},$$

is the health gains displaced to finance the additional costs of financing Araamax over each of the two periods $\left(2f_1\overline{\Delta E}_1\right)$ by displacing services with an aICER of m.

The Institution's payoff to reimbursing Araamax in Period 2, then Araamaxplus in Period 3 (action Reimburse, R, only) is:

$$\Delta E = \left(\overline{\Delta E}_1 - \frac{f_1\overline{\Delta E}_1}{m}\right) + \left(\overline{\Delta E}_1 + \overline{\Delta E}_2 - \frac{f_1\overline{\Delta E}_1}{m} - \frac{f_2\overline{\Delta E}_2}{m}\right),$$

where:

$$\overline{\Delta E}_1 - \frac{f_1\overline{\Delta E}_1}{m}$$

is the net health effect for the population from reimbursing Araamax in Period 2, compared with continuing to reimburse Rathmab and:

$$\overline{\Delta E}_1 + \overline{\Delta E}_2 - \frac{f_1\overline{\Delta E}_1}{m} - \frac{f_2\overline{\Delta E}_2}{m}$$

is the net health effect for the population from financing Araamaxplus in Period 3 compared with the health that would have occurred if the Institution continued to finance Rathmab.

10.4.2.3   Parameters, Variables and Conditions

- $\overline{\mathcal{R}}$ is the Firm's fixed cost for developing and trialling a new drug. It is the same for both drugs.
- $\overline{\Delta E}_1$ is the additional health effect of Araamax compared with Rathmab.
- $\overline{\Delta E}_2$ is the additional health effect of Araamaxplus compared with Araamax.
- m is the aICER of the services of the least cost-effective existing programme in contraction, which is optimally displaced in order to finance the additional cost of the new drug Araamax in Periods 2 and 3.
- c_1 is the IMER (compared with Rathmab) of producing Araamax.
- c_2 is the IMER (compared with Rathmab) of producing Araamaxplus.
- f_1 is the IPER of Araamax compared with Rathmab.
- f_2 is the IPER of Araamaxplus compared with Araamax.

The parameters and variables that describe the payoffs of the actions available to the Institution can be specified in terms of the total cost and unit cost of achieving them.

-

$$\frac{f_j \overline{\Delta E_j}}{m}$$

– is the health effects displaced if the additional cost of the additional health gains $\left(\frac{f_j \overline{\Delta E_j}}{m}\right)$ are financed by displacing services with an aICER of m, where $j = 1$ or 2 and refers to the IPERs of the two drugs.

10.4.2.4 Conditions

- There is no uncertainty in the value of any parameters and variables at any stage in the Game for either player.
- The discount rate is zero.
- The Firm is efficient in its R&D process; there is no way of trialling and developing a new drug that would reduce the fixed costs of R&D.
-

$$\overline{\Delta E}_1, \overline{\Delta E}_2 > 0.$$

– The drugs brought to the Institution are clinically innovative. This is, they have a clinical advantage compared with the best available existing therapy for the target group of patients. The clinical innovation is constant for the identified group of target patients, and is known with certainty.

- $d = m > 0.$

– The aICER of the services displaced to finance the additional financial costs of the new drug is greater than zero. It is also the least cost-effective of all existing options to contract programmes (efficient displacement), therefore $\beta_c = m.$

- $\Delta E^D > 0.$

– It follows from $m > 0$ that displacing services to finance the additional costs of the new drug will lead to a loss in health effects for patients who would otherwise have received these services.

- ΔE^D is continuous.

– The funding to the displaced services can be reduced or increased by the smallest increment. If the funding is changed, the effect will change in the same direction.

- $f_1, f_2 > 0$

– The price per additional effect of the new drug compared with the best available therapy is greater than 0.

- $c_1 > c_2 > 0$

  - The IMER (compared with Rathmab) of Araamax is c_1. ($5,000(j)$ Table 10.4) The IMER (compared to Rathmab) of Araamaxplus is c_2. ($2,176(n)$ Table 10.4) The total cost of producing a vial of Araamaxplus is higher than for Araamax, which is in turn higher than for a vial of Rathmab. ($250 (c) < $500(c) < $650(h)$ Table 10.2). The technique of producing Araamax was fundamentally different to that of producing a vial of Rathmab, which accounts for the significantly higher cost of production per vial.
  - However, the slightly more complex technique required to produce the more clinically effective version of the drug Araamax increases the overall cost only slightly, hence the IMER of Araamax (for the incremental health compared with Rathmab) is higher than that for Araamaxplus (for the incremental health gains compared with Rathmab). Araamaxplus contains innovation in manufacturing as well as clinical innovation.

10.5   Theory Proper

We assume that the Firm will select its strategy by maximising its economic rent and the Institution will select its strategies so as to maximise the npvPH from the current and future budgets.

10.6   Solution

We use backward induction to solve the game.

10.6.1   Stage 6

In Stage 6, the Institution can choose to Reimburse Araamaxplus at the offer price or continue to purchase Araamax at the prevailing price. Its decision rule is to select the action Reimburse (R) if the payoff is greater than or equal to the payoff to continuing to purchase Araamax (C). These payoffs are presented in Fig. 10.1.

$$\left(\overline{\Delta E}_1 - \frac{f_1 \overline{\Delta E}_1}{m}\right) + \left(\overline{\Delta E}_1 + \overline{\Delta E}_2 - \frac{f_2 \overline{\Delta E}_1}{m} - \frac{f_1 \overline{\Delta E}_2}{m}\right) \geq 2\overline{\Delta E}_1 - \frac{2f_1 \overline{\Delta E}_1}{m}$$

$$\Rightarrow \overline{\Delta E}_2 - \frac{f_2 \overline{\Delta E}_2}{m} \geq 0$$

$$\Rightarrow (m - f_2) \geq 0$$

$$\Rightarrow m \geq f_2.$$

This decision rule can be expressed in words as: if the IPER of the future drug Araamaxplus (calculated relative to Araamax) is less than or equal to the aICER of displaced services, the Institution will reimburse the future drug.

10.6.2 Stage 5

In Stage 5, the Firm chooses to price the future drug $f_2 = m$ because if it reduces the price below this IPER it will not sell a greater quantity of the drug and if it prices higher it will not sell any of the drug. This characteristic is a consequence of both the decision rule that the Reimburser is required to follow at indifference between Reimbursement and the best alternative strategy and the discrete nature of the policy to reimburse a new drug in a universal health care system.

Therefore:

$$f_2 = m \tag{10.3}$$

10.6.3 Stage 4

In Stage 4, the Firm makes the decision to either: (1) manufacture and sell Araamax and also develop the second drug, Araamaxplus; or (2) only manufacture and sell Araamax. The Firm will choose to invest a second fixed budget into R&D if the payoff from investing in the second drug's development is greater than the payoff from manufacture of Araamax only. These payoffs are presented in Fig. 10.1.

$$\left(f_1 \overline{\Delta E}_1 - c_1 \overline{\Delta E}_1 - \mathcal{R}\right) + \left(f_1 \overline{\Delta E}_1 + f_2 \overline{\Delta E}_2 - c_2\left(\overline{\Delta E}_1 + \overline{\Delta E}_2\right) - \mathcal{R}\right) \geq 2f_1 \overline{\Delta E}_1 - 2c_1 \overline{\Delta E}_1 - \mathcal{R}$$

$$\Rightarrow f_2 \overline{\Delta E}_2 - c_2\left(\overline{\Delta E}_1 + \overline{\Delta E}_2\right) + c_1 \overline{\Delta E}_1 - \mathcal{R} \geq 0$$

$$\Rightarrow \overline{\Delta E}_2(f_2 - c_2) + \overline{\Delta E}_1(c_1 - c_2) - \mathcal{R} \geq 0 \tag{10.4}$$

The economic profit from the sale of the additional health effects of Araamaxplus compared with Araamax is:

$$\overline{\Delta E}_2(f_2 - c_2),$$

and the savings that come from selling the health gains of Araamax relative to Rathmab at the same price but at a lower a IMER:

$$\overline{\Delta E}_1(c_1 - c_2),$$

must outweigh the additional costs of R&D. However, from Eq. (10.3) we know that:

$$f_2 = m.$$

So we can substitute this result into Eq. (10.4). Therefore if the following condition applies:

$$\overline{\Delta E}_2(m - c_2) + \overline{\Delta E}_1(c_1 - c_2) \geq \overline{\mathcal{R}}, \tag{10.5}$$

then the Firm will choose to develop the second drug. (We assume that the Firm will invest in R&D for Araamaxplus if it is indifferent between this action and the action of manufacture only.)

If the following condition applies,

$$\overline{\Delta E}_2(m - c_2) + \overline{\Delta E}_1(c_1 - c_2) < \overline{\mathcal{R}}, \tag{10.6}$$

then the Firm will choose not to develop Araamaxplus because the additional costs of R&D $\left(\overline{\mathcal{R}}\right)$ are greater than the two sources of gains to the Firm from development:

- The additional economic rent $(m - c_2)$ from the additional units of health effects that can be sold $\left(\overline{\Delta E_2}\right)$; and
- The reduction in the cost per effect of producing the units $\overline{\Delta E_1}$ which occurs because $c_1 > c_2$.

Finally, the following exogenous parameters drive this decision: $\overline{\Delta E_1}$, $\overline{\Delta E_2}$ m, c_1, c_2 and $\mathcal{R}$.

Stage 4 highlights that the opportunity for the Firm to generate innovation in the manufacturing process is a driver of investment in R&D, in addition to the opportunity to generate clinical innovation.

10.6.4 Stage 3

The Institution chooses to Reimburse the new drug Araamax or do Nothing in Stage 3. The payoff to this decision depends upon the Firm's decision in Stage 4.[6]

10.6.4.1 Araamaxplus Is Not Produced in Stage 4

From Eq. (10.6), if:

$$\overline{\Delta E_2}(m - c_2) + \overline{\Delta E_1}(c_1 - c_2) < \overline{\mathcal{R}},$$

then the Firm will not produce the second drug, Araamaxplus, hence the payoff to the Institution's decision to reimburse Araamax if the second drug is not produced is:

$$\Delta E = 2\overline{\Delta E_1} - \frac{2f_1\overline{\Delta E_1}}{m}.$$

Therefore the decision rule is that the Institution will Reimburse if:

$$2\overline{\Delta E_1} - \frac{2f_1\overline{\Delta E_1}}{m} \geq 0$$
$$\Rightarrow m - f_1 \geq 0$$
$$\Rightarrow m \geq f_1.$$

Hence, if the Institution anticipates that the Firm will choose not to develop the second drug Araamaxplus, then the Institution will choose to reimburse Araamax if the IPER of Araamax versus Rathmab is less than or equal to the aICER of displaced services.

10.6.4.2 Araamaxplus Is Produced in Stage 4

However, from Eq. (10.6) if:

$$\overline{\Delta E_2}(m - c_2) + \overline{\Delta E_1}(c_1 - c_2) \geq \overline{\mathcal{R}},$$

then the Firm will produce the second drug and the Institution's payoff to reimbursing Araamax is:

---

[6] The reason that the Institution can anticipate the outcome of Stage 4 when the Game is at Stage 3 is because all information is in the public domain, the motivations for players are in the public domain and each player makes decisions that take into account the other Player's responses. This is effectively the rationale for solving this game using backward induction.

$$\Delta E = \left(\overline{\Delta E_1} - \frac{f_1 \overline{\Delta E_1}}{m} \right) + \left(\overline{\Delta E_1} + \overline{\Delta E_2} - \frac{f_1 \overline{\Delta E_1}}{m} - \frac{f_2 \overline{\Delta E_2}}{m} \right).$$

Therefore the decision rule is to reimburse the drug at the offer price if:

$$\left(\overline{\Delta E_1} - \frac{f_1 \overline{\Delta E_1}}{m} \right) + \left(\overline{\Delta E_1} + \overline{\Delta E_2} - \frac{f_1 \overline{\Delta E_1}}{m} - \frac{f_2 \overline{\Delta E_2}}{m} \right) \geq 0$$

$$\Rightarrow 2\overline{\Delta E_1} + \overline{\Delta E_2} - \frac{2f_1 \overline{\Delta E_1}}{m} - \frac{f_2 \overline{\Delta E_2}}{m} \geq 0,$$

but from Stage 5 we have the result that $m = f_2$

$$\therefore 2\overline{\Delta E_1} + \overline{\Delta E_2} - \frac{2f_1 \overline{\Delta E_1}}{m} - \overline{\Delta E_2} \geq 0$$

$$\Rightarrow 2\overline{\Delta E_1} - \frac{2f_1 \overline{\Delta E_1}}{m} \geq 0$$

$$\Rightarrow 2d - 2f_1 \geq 0$$
$$\Rightarrow m \geq f_1.$$

Therefore, if the Firm will not produce Araamaxplus, then the Institution anticipates this action (best response and complete and perfect information) and provided that $m \geq f_1$ it will reimburse Araamax.

10.6.4.3   Result of Stage 3

Regardless of whether the Firm will choose to develop the second drug in Stage 4, the Institution will only reimburse Araamax if the IPER is less than or equal to the aICER of the displaced services.

10.6.5   Stage 2

In Stage 2 the Firm will choose to price the new drug and it will choose a price so as to maximise economic rent. This will occur when $f_1 = m$. Above this price there will be no sales and at a lower price there will be no increase in sales.

10.6.6   Stage 1

In Stage 1, the Firm chooses to invest in the R&D for Araamax or do nothing. If the Firm does Nothing, the game ends.

The payoff to R&D for Araamax depends upon whether or not the exogenous parameters:: $\overline{\Delta E_1}, \overline{\Delta E_2}, m, c_1, c_2$ and $\mathcal{R}$ are such that the Firm has an incentive to invest in the development of Araamaxplus, the second new drug.

Firm has Incentive to Develop Araamaxplus in Stage 4.

If the Firm has an incentive to develop the second drug rather than manufacture and develop only the first drug, then the Firm's payoff to Development in Stage 1 is:

$$\pi = m\overline{\Delta E_1} - c_1\overline{\Delta E_1} - \overline{\mathcal{R}}.$$

Therefore, the Firm's decision rule is to invest in R&D if the payoff to Develop is greater than the payoff to do Nothing:

$$\left(f_1\overline{\Delta E_1} - c_1\overline{\Delta E_1} - \overline{\mathcal{R}}\right) + \left(f_1\overline{\Delta E_1} + f_2\overline{\Delta E_2} - c_2\left(\overline{\Delta E_1} + \overline{\Delta E_2}\right) - \overline{\mathcal{R}}\right) \geq 0,$$

where

$$f_2 = f_1 = m$$
$$\therefore \left(m\overline{\Delta E_1} - c_1\overline{\Delta E_1} - \overline{\mathcal{R}}\right) + \left(m\overline{\Delta E_1} + d\overline{\Delta E_2} - c_2\left(\overline{\Delta E_1} + \overline{\Delta E_2}\right) - \overline{\mathcal{R}}\right) \geq 0$$
$$\Rightarrow 2m\overline{\Delta E_1} + m\overline{\Delta E_2} \geq c_2\left(\overline{\Delta E_1} + \overline{\Delta E_2}\right) + c_1\overline{\Delta E_1} + 2\overline{\mathcal{R}}$$
$$\Rightarrow m\left(2\overline{\Delta E_1} + \overline{\Delta E_2}\right) \geq c_2\left(\overline{\Delta E_1} + \overline{\Delta E_2}\right) + c_1\overline{\Delta E_1} + 2\overline{\mathcal{R}}.$$

$$(10.7)$$

That is, the Firm will invest in the Development of Araamax in Period 1 if the revenue from the clinical innovation over the two periods:

$$m\left(2\overline{\Delta E_1} + \overline{\Delta E_2}\right)$$

is greater than the cost of developing and manufacturing the two drugs:

$$c_2\left(\overline{\Delta E_1} + \overline{\Delta E_2}\right) + c_1\overline{\Delta E_1} + 2\overline{\mathcal{R}}.$$

Otherwise the Firm will choose to do Nothing.

10.6.6.1   Firm Has No Incentive to Invest in the Second Drug

If the Firm will not invest in the second drug, then the payoff to the Firm from choosing to Develop the first drug rather than do Nothing is:

$$2f_1\overline{\Delta E_1} - 2c_1\overline{\Delta E_1} - \overline{\mathcal{R}} > 0.$$

Hence, if the following condition is met

$$2\overline{\Delta E_1}(m - c_1) - \overline{\mathcal{R}} > 0, \tag{10.8}$$

then the Firm will develop the first drug, Araamax, but not Araamaxplus. That is, the Firm will Develop and Manufacture Araamax if the additional economic rent on the total units sold at an IPER of f_1 and produced at an IMER of c_1 is greater than the cost of R&D. Otherwise, the Firm will do Nothing.

10.6.7   Equilibrium Outcomes

There are three possible equilibrium outcomes: (i) no drugs are produced; (ii) only Araamax is produced; and (iii) both Araamax and Araamaxplus are produced.

The equilibrium price under scenarios (ii) and (iii) is m, the threshold IPER. There is no increase in the health of the population relative to scenario (i) under either scenario (ii) or scenario (iii). The Firm's profit will depend upon the scenario. If there had been existing inefficiency in the health care budget, then there would have been a gain in health effects for the population under scenarios (ii) and (iii). However, this would have been as a consequence of the budget being inefficient initially and the allocative inefficiency reduced. The same health gain for the population could have been achieved by a process such as PBMA.

The gain in social welfare is given by the combined payoffs of the Firm and the Institution. The entire economic value of the surplus is appropriated by the Firm as a consequence of the profit-maximising choice of offer price by the Firm and the rule that requires the Institution to Reimburse the new drug if $f \le \beta_c$.

10.7   Discussion

The equilibrium IPER of the two drugs (Araamax and Araamaxplus) is the same; it is the Institution's reimbursement threshold price, which for this Institution is β_c with a quantitative value of m. It is the same as the equilibrium price in Games 1 and 2.

10.7.1 Is a Premium a Necessary or Sufficient Condition for Investment in a Future Drug?

> A premium is neither a necessary nor a sufficient condition for the Firm to invest in a future drug.

The *premium* on the current drug is *not a sufficient condition* because the decision for the Firm to invest in R&D for the both drugs is a function of a number of parameters, only one of which is the IPER of the future drug, and even with a premium there may be no incentive to invest, for example if $c_2 \gg c_1$. The other parameters that this decision is a function of, and that are specified in the Game are:

- $\overline{\mathcal{R}}$, the fixed cost of R&D;
- c_2 and c_1 the costs of manufacturing the drugs expressed as IMERs, relative to the IPER;
- The difference in the IMERs of the two drugs (innovation in manufacturing, $c_2 - c_1 > 0$); and
- The clinical innovation of the drugs relative to the best available therapy ΔE_1 and ΔE_2

> **Note**
> We have assumed that the information about the future costs of manufacture and all other parameters are known with certainty and are public information. This is unrealistic and the implications of relaxing this assumption are set out in the discussion.

The *premium* is *not a necessary condition* because the Firm has an incentive to invest in R&D for the second drug even without the premium in Period 2 for Araamax, provided that the above parameters meet the requirements set out in Stage 4 and Stage 1. Other factors that influence the decision to invest in R&D are not included in the Game: competition from me-too drugs and development of alternative non-pharmaco-therapies are examples.

The Institution is indifferent between the three outcomes of the game (no drugs, one drug or two drugs), because there is no increase in the population's health as a consequence of any outcome. Had allocative inefficiency been an initial condition, the health of the population would have increased, but there would be no net economic benefit from reimbursement; the health benefit was a consequence of improving overall efficiency and this could have been achieved by reallocation.

In conclusion, there is no price above β_c whereby the npvPH is increased, hence there is no incentive for the Institution to pay a premium for Araamax in Period 2. Any premium will represent a loss to the Institution because the Firm prices the future drug at β_c and hence there is no mechanism whereby the Institution can recoup the health gains foregone in Period 2.

However, this result does not necessarily mean that there is no economic justification for pricing above β_c in Period 2. Some economists could argue that maximising social welfare (economic rent plus consumer welfare) is society's objective whereas maximising consumer welfare (increase in population health) is the Institution's objective. The two are not necessarily consistent.

10.7.2 Is There a Situation Whereby a Premium for Araamax in Period 2 Will Increase Social Welfare?

Is it possible that the Institution's decision to not price above β_c in Period 2, in order to maximise the npvPH from this and future budgets, is at the cost of social welfare? The possibility of this outcome can be inferred from Santerre and Vernon (2006). These authors found that every dollar invested by consumers in pharmaceutical R&D via higher prices for drugs over the period 1960 to 2000 led to an additional $28 in social welfare (consumer welfare plus economic rent).[7] Assume that Santerre and Vernon's result is an accurate estimate of the ratio intended by the authors. The result cannot tell us whether consumers have recouped their initial investment or whether the entire social welfare was appropriated by the firm and the consumers have a net loss in consumer welfare. But Santerre and Vernon do not comment on this issue. This lack of comment could signal a difference in the US approach to health economics compared with the rest of the OECD. Maybe in the US, economists would argue that the allocation of this gain in social welfare across producers and consumers is irrelevant; what matters is that the social welfare is maximised.

In terms of the Game presented in this chapter, this position would mean that an outcome that results in maximising the net present value of social welfare (npvSW) is preferable to the outcome that maximises the net present value of population's health (npvPH) but at a lower npvSW.

The possibility that the equilibrium outcome of the Game presented in this chapter could be maximising npvPH at the cost of maximising npvSW cannot be excluded. Hence the following question:

Is it possible that in seeking to maximise npvPH, the Reimburser makes a decision in Period 2 that maximises npvPH over the three periods but does not maximise npvSW over these periods?

---

[7] The reasons why this return is likely to be a significant overestimate of the ratio intended by the authors are discussed in Pekarsky (2012, Appendix 1). The reasons why the ratio intended by the authors could result in an overestimate of the ratio of interest to a country with a fixed or constrained budget are discussed in Chaps. 1 and 3 and also Pekarsky (2012, Appendix 2). In short, it does not consider the allocation of surplus between the firm and consumers.

First we establish the necessary and/or sufficient conditions under which this situation would occur. Then we establish the changes in the Game that would have to occur in order for the production of the second drug to occur and the npvSW to be maximised.

10.7.2.1 Conditions

Two equations are used to define the conditions that correspond to the problem of nonproduction of Araamaxplus at an IPER $=m$ for Araamax in Period 2 but production of Araamaxplus if there were a premium for Araamax over β_c in Period 2.

- The Firm cannot finance the production of the second drug from the economic rent available from the first drug in Period 2.

$$\overline{\Delta E_1}(m - c_1) < \overline{\mathcal{R}}. \tag{10.9}$$

where $m - c_1$ is the economic rent received on each incremental health effect sold in Period 2.
- There is a price above β_c, which is $\beta_c + \gamma$, at which the Firm can finance the R&D.

$$\overline{\Delta E_1}(m + \gamma - c_1) = \overline{\mathcal{R}},$$

which can be rearranged as:

$$\gamma = \frac{\overline{\mathcal{R}}}{\overline{\Delta E_1}} + c_1 - m. \tag{10.10}$$

Now we determine the conditions under which the following scenario occurs:
- The social welfare is maximised if both drugs are produced, and the above two conditions [Eq. (10.9) and Eq. (10.10)] apply.

The approach we take is to apply the strong and weak compensation tests.[8] The formal definitions of the terms strong and weak compensation tests are set out in Mas-Colell et al. (1995 pp. 829–831) and discussed in Pekarsky (2012, Appendix 9).

---

[8] In simple terms the strong compensation test means that the policy of a premium in the situation specified by Eq. (10.9) and Eq. (10.11) will always result in a gain in npvSW—the gain in economic rent in Period 3 to the Firm is greater that the loss to consumers in Period 2. In this case, policy of a premium always passes the hypothetical compensation test. If only the weak compensation test is met, then the hypothetical compensation test can be passed by the policy conditionally only. [For a more extensive discussion see Pekarsky (2012, Appendix 9)].

10.7.2.2   Applying the Hypothetical Compensation Test

Our starting point is the observation that there is a loss to the Institution if it chooses to reimburse the new drug at an IPER above m in Period 1. This loss is given in terms of units of health and is:

$$Loss = \frac{\gamma \overline{\Delta E_1}}{m}. \tag{10.11}$$

This is the health gains forgone due to the additional expenditure (the premium) on the sale of each unit of clinical innovation from Araamax.

The hypothetical compensation test is passed if, under the scenario defined by conditions (1) and (2) above, the gain in producer's surplus as a consequence of producing two drugs rather than one drug is greater than the amount that would be required to be paid by the Firm to the Institution to compensate for the loss in Period 2. If this test can be passed for all values of relevant parameters then the strong compensation test is passed. If the hypothetical compensation is conditional on values of the relevant parameters, then only the weak compensation test applies.

From Eq. (10.11) we see that the amount that the Firm would need to pay the Institution to compensate them for the loss is:

$$\gamma \overline{\Delta E_1}$$

The additional producer's surplus in Period 3 from producing two drugs rather than one drug is given by the difference in the Firm's payoff in Period 3 under the two scenarios. The difference in the economic rent in Period 3 can be derived from Eq. (10.1) and Eq. (10.2).

$$\begin{aligned} \Delta \pi_3 &= \left(f_1 \overline{\Delta E_1} + f_2 \overline{\Delta E_2} - c_2 \left(\overline{\Delta E_1} + \overline{\Delta E_2} \right) \right) - \left(f_1 \overline{\Delta E_1} - c_1 \overline{\Delta E_1} \right) \\ &= f_2 \overline{\Delta E_2} - c_2 \overline{\Delta E_1} - c_2 \overline{\Delta E_2} + c_1 \overline{\Delta E_1} \\ &= \overline{\Delta E_2} (f_2 - c_2) + \overline{\Delta E_1} (c_1 - c_2). \end{aligned}$$

This is the additional economic rent $(f_2 - c_2)$ on the sales of the clinically innovative units of Araamaxplus plus the additional economic rent due to the reduced cost of producing $(c_1 - c_2)$ the clinically innovative units first developed with Araamax $\overline{\Delta E_1}$.

Now we need to find the conditions under which:

$$\overline{\Delta E_2} (f_2 - c_2) + \overline{\Delta E_1} (c_1 - c_2) > \gamma \overline{\Delta E_1}. \tag{10.12}$$

Now $f_2 = m$, that is, the IPER in Period 3 for the future drug Araamaxplus is β_c which has a quantitative value of m. That is, we are assuming the compensation is separate from any payment related to the purchase of the new drug.

Furthermore,

$$\overline{\Delta E_2} = \kappa \overline{\Delta E_1} > 0,$$

where $\overline{\Delta E_1} \kappa > 0$.

That is, the clinical innovation of Araamaxplus relative to Araamax can be expressed as a linear function of clinical innovation of Araamax relative to Rathmab. $\overline{\Delta E_2}$ can be less than or greater than $\overline{\Delta E_1}$ but must be greater than zero.

Therefore we substitute this relationship into Eq. (10.12):

$$\kappa \overline{\Delta E_1}(m - c_2) + \overline{\Delta E_1}(c_1 - c_2) > \gamma \overline{\Delta E_1}.$$

Now $\overline{\Delta E_1} > 0$, therefore we can divide through to obtain the conditions under which the hypothetical compensation test can be met:

$$\kappa(m - c_2) + (c_1 - c_2) > \gamma, \tag{10.13}$$

where the first term is the economic rent on clinically innovative units and the second term is the economic rent due to manufacturing innovation. This condition means that in order to compensate the Institution for their loss in Period 2, the Firm requires sufficient additional economic rent from Period 3, where this rent is sourced from economic rent on clinically innovative units of Araamaxplus and manufacturing innovation on clinically innovative units of Araamax.

We can derive a second alternative expression for this condition. From Eq. (10.10):

$$\gamma = \frac{\overline{\mathcal{R}}}{\overline{\Delta E_1}} + c_1 - m,$$

which we substitute into Eq. (10.13):

$$\kappa(m - c_2) + (c_1 - c_2) > \frac{\overline{\mathcal{R}}}{\overline{\Delta E_1}} + c_1 - m$$

$$\Rightarrow \kappa(m - c_2) - c_2 + m > \frac{\overline{\mathcal{R}}}{\overline{\Delta E_1}}$$

$$\Rightarrow (\kappa + 1)(m - c_2) > \frac{\overline{\mathcal{R}}}{\overline{\Delta E_1}}.$$

The second (alternative) expression of the condition for the compensation test is saying that the additional economic rent on every additional innovative health effect of Araamaxplus compared to Rathmab (the existing drug), must be greater than the cost of R&D per incremental health effect of Araamax compared with Rathmab.

10.7.2.3 Results of the Hypothetical Compensation Test

The first result is that the hypothetical compensation test can be passed conditionally, but not unconditionally. The strong (unconditional) compensation test cannot be passed because there are values of κ, c_1, c_2, ΔE_1, $\mathcal{R}$, and m such that the additional premium, even though it will produce an additional drug, will result in a net reduction in social welfare. Similarly, the weak compensation test can be passed because these parameters can take values that result in a net social welfare gain as a consequence of the premium compared with the situation of no premium. What this means is that if the conditions in Eq. (10.9) and Eq. (10.10) are met, using a premium will result in Araamaxplus being produced but this will only lead to an increase in npvSW under certain conditions, as outlined in Eq. (10.14).

The second result is that regardless of whether the compensation test is passed, the Firm will be better off if a premium is paid for two reasons. First, it maintains a share of the additional premium paid in Period 2 as economic rent. This is because less than 30 % is allocated to NME R&D under current conditions (Reinhardt 2007); this amount could change if those conditions were changed. Second, the Firm is in receipt of any additional economic rent from the future drug, which it would not have been in receipt of otherwise; if there is no actual compensation, it will maintain this rent.

10.7.2.4 Necessary and Sufficient Conditions for the Premium Policy to Pass the Compensation Test

Now we can determine the necessary and sufficient conditions for there to be a gain in the npvSW and hence pass the weak compensation test. Of particular interest in the PEND is the role of the clinical innovation of the future drug in these conditions. Is clinical innovation either a necessary or sufficient condition, or is it neither?

First, Eq. (10.13) and its alternative expression, Eq. (10.14), set out the necessary conditions for the policy of paying a premium when there is no incentive for the Firm to invest in R&D in Period 2, because the funds are not available from internal funds (economic rent) in Period 2.

Second, from Eq. (10.13) and Eq. (10.14) we can see that even if there is no clinical innovation in the second drug, ($\kappa = 0$), there is still an opportunity for there to be a gain in social welfare that could pass the hypothetical compensation test. That is, there exist values of the parameters c_1, c_2, ΔE_1, $\mathcal{R}$, and m such that the Institution can be compensated even if there is no clinical innovation. One example is significant manufacturing innovation, characterised by $c_1 - c_2 > 0$. Therefore, the existence of clinical innovation for Araamaxplus is not a necessary condition for there to be a net gain in social welfare as a consequence of the premium and the second drug.

Third, we can also see from Eq. (10.13) and Eq. (10.14) that even if there is clinical innovation ($\theta > 0$), there are values κ, c_1, c_2, ΔE_1, $\mathcal{R}$, and m such that there is a net loss in social welfare by producing the second drug. For example, in Eq. (10.14), even if $\kappa \gg 0$, if the cost of manufacturing these incremental gains is more than the cost of purchasing them within existing technologies, there is a net social welfare loss. Even if $m > c_2$, if the cost of R&D ($\mathcal{R}$) is too high, the situation fails the hypothetical compensation test. Therefore, the existence of clinical innovation in Araamaxplus is not a sufficient condition for the post-premium world to pass either the strong or weak compensation test.

In conclusion, even if there were a premium that could be paid above β_c that would result in innovation that would otherwise not occur, then this result, an additional future drug, is neither necessary nor sufficient for there to be a net increase in social welfare; the strong compensation test is not passed by the policy of a premium over β_c. Furthermore, clinical innovation of the future drug (Araamaxplus) relative to the new drug (Araamax) is neither a necessary nor sufficient condition for this to occur, regardless of the extent of this innovation. Manufacturing innovation and more efficient R&D are also drivers of the net social welfare benefit. Furthermore, the analysis above assumes that all internal funds generated by the premium are allocated to R&D for the future drug. If we were to take into account the evidence that only a proportion of internal funds are invested in NME R&D, possibly less than 30 % (Reinhardt 2007), then this would make it less likely that there will be sufficient future rent to compensate the Institution, whose foregone benefit per additional future drug will be higher as a result.

However, the analysis did identify situations where the payment of this premium does result in a net gain in social welfare; cases where the conditions in are Eq. (10.14) met and the weak compensation test is passed. It is possible that pursuing a strategy to maximise the npvPH can be at the cost of npvSW? What should the Institution do in this case?

10.7.2.5 What Incentives Are Required for the Institution to Agree to Price Above the Equilibrium Price in Period 1?

As the Game is specified currently, there is no incentive for the Institution to price above $\beta_c = m$ in Period 2. This is because even if this results in a net social welfare gain (the conditions in Eq. (10.13) are met), if no compensation occurs there is a net reduction in the population's health. There is no incentive for the Institution to pay a premium.

At this point there are two options for taking the analysis forward: (1) to adopt the premium policy, conditionally and accept the final division of social surplus across the consumers and the producers (no actual compensation) or (2) to generate a situation in which there is actual compensation.

Under the first option we could argue that this result (if the premium is not paid the npvSW is reduced) is proof that there are conditions under which there is a deadweight social loss to price control. [See Pekarsky (2012, Appendix 7)].

Therefore, the Institution should accept that maximising social welfare is the relevant test and accept an outcome of lower npvPH but higher npvSW (economic rent plus health). However, given that the scenario above passed only the weak compensation test, it would be necessary for the Firm to demonstrate that the conditions in Eq. (10.13) are met for a particular future drug. If these conditions are not met the premium will result in an additional drug and increased economic rent but less npvPH and less npvSW. Whether or not the Firm is able to demonstrate that these conditions are met is unclear, given the uncertainty associated with the characteristics of future drugs. What is even less likely is that consumers and policy makers will accept this result of reduced npvPH and higher npvSW, even if this outcome is apparently acceptable to US pharma-economists such as Santerre and Vernon.

Significantly, even if the Firm is able to demonstrate that these conditions are met, then the outcome of worse health and more social welfare is particularly difficult to defend. The political reason is that even though some economists might argue it is an acceptable outcome, the entire PEND is premised on the position that higher prices are a win-win situation—more for the firm and more for the population's health. The economic reason is that when there is an opportunity for any surplus to be shared between the producer and consumers via a lower price for the future drug, then what is stopping the compensation from actually occurring and making all parties better off? This is particularly the case when it is the Institution not the Firm that has taken on the costs (and risks) of financing R&D. Hence the first option, to adopt the policy of a premium conditionally and accept the final allocation of surplus without actual compensation, is unlikely to be acceptable.

The second option is that, if the conditions in Eq. (10.13) are met, we could generate an incentive for the Institution to pay this premium despite the short-term reduction in health. This incentive is achieved by the Firm offering a contract to the Institution for it to be able to recoup its up-front additional costs in Period 2. This in turn leads to the result from Chap. 9: the Firm would prefer to contract with a Bank if the Institution is risk-averse relative to the Bank and requires appropriate compensation for the risky investment in Firm R&D. The question of whether the Firm can demonstrate that these conditions can be met prior to the final clinical trials of the drug remains a significant barrier to such a contract.

In summary, even though there are conditions under which paying a premium for a current drug will lead to an additional future drug and a net gain in social welfare, Institutions need an incentive to provide this premium. It is unlikely that a Firm can demonstrate that the conditions under which this premium can result in a net increase in social welfare are met with sufficient certainty. Even less likely is the acceptance of a policy such as that proposed by Jena and Philipson whereby all new drugs are provided with a premium, regardless of whether the conditions in Eq. (10.13) are met. In this case, the only certain result is the increased economic rent in that period from the additional premium.

10.8 Conclusion

The Reimburser revisits her question.

1. How should the Institution respond to the following Threat?

> When the Institution buys this new drug, it buys the health effects from this drug and the health benefits from future innovation. This is not the case with other health programmes. Therefore, unless the Institution pays a premium for the health effects from the new drug, the population will be worse off because innovation will be suboptimal and the future drug will not be produced.

(a) The existence of a premium for the current drug is neither a necessary nor sufficient condition for there to be an incentive for the Firm to produce a future drug.

(b) If there exists a situation in which a premium is necessary to produce a second drug and the premium is paid, then the development of this future drug is not a sufficient condition for this to action to result in a net increase in npvSW (the increase in economic rent plus the increase in future consumer welfare net the loss from reduced health today).

(c) The existence of clinical innovation in the future drug, regardless of the size of this innovation, is neither a necessary nor sufficient condition for the hypothetical compensation test to be passed. However, for a given IMER and IPER, the greater the clinical innovation the greater the surplus, all of which is appropriated by the Firm if the IPER $= \beta_c$.

(d) If the conditions are met such that the weak hypothetical compensation test can be passed by the policy of a premium, then the Firm should generate an incentive for the Institution to provide the premium. This incentive would be achieved by the Firm contracting to provide the Institution with a share of the future drug's surplus, including the value of manufacturing as well as clinical surplus. However, the information required to demonstrate that the conditions for passing the compensation test are passed is unlikely to be available prior to the drug's development.

The Reimburser asks the Firm for proof that the conditions for passing the compensation test are met by the premium payment for Araamax. The Firm provides her with the following evidence: (1) they cannot fund Araamax's development without the premium; (2) they can fund it with the premium; and (3) Araamax will be highly clinically innovative. The Reimburser points out that this is not sufficient for the Firm to guarantee that the hypothetical compensation test is passed.

The Reimburser explains to the Firm that she would prefer that they approach the Capital Market for the additional funds that they require in order to develop Araamaxplus. The Institution cannot bear the risks that arise from being uncertain about the value of parameters such as the level of manufacturing innovation of the future drug and the costs of R&D, both of which are private information for the Firm (not in the public domain). The Firm responds by providing an excerpt from the Congressional Budget Office Report on Research and Development in the Pharmaceutical industry (US Congressional Budget Office 2006).

> A relatively close relationship exists between drug firms' current R&D spending and current sales revenue for two reasons. First, successful new drugs generate large cash flows that can be invested in R&D (their manufacturing costs are usually very low relative to their price). Second, alternative sources of investment capital—from the bond and stock markets—are not perfect substitutes for cash flow financing. Those alternative sources of capital are more expensive because lenders and prospective new shareholders require compensation (in the form of higher returns) for the additional risk they bear compared with the firm, which has more information about the drug under development, its current status, and its ultimate chance of success. (p. 9)

The Reimburser asks the Firm whether it believes that the Institution does not need to be compensated for its investment of "large cash flows" (foregone health). After all, the Institution has not been provided with this information either. The Firm responds that patients benefit from the new drugs, but the Capital Market does not. The Reimburser points out that the price that she pays for the health effect of new drugs is the same price as what she could use to purchase health gains from existing technologies (IPER $= \beta_c$). There is no economic benefit to the population from purchasing at the health shadow price.

Then the Reimburser asks: What is this information? How can the Firm have this information about future costs and effect before they start the clinical trials? The Firm assures the Reimburser that they have this information. The Reimburser offers to act as a knowledge broker and explain this information to the Capital Market, provided that the Institution can see this information first.

References

Chen Y-F, Jobanputra P, Barton P, Jowett S, Bryan S, Clark W, Fry-Smith A, Burls A, 42 (2006) A systematic review of the effectiveness of adalimumab, etanercept and infliximab for the treatment of rheumatoid arthritis in adults and an economic evaluation of their cost-effectiveness. Health Technol Assess 10:1–229, iii-iv, xi-xiii

Congressional Budget Office US (2006) Research and development in the pharmaceutical industry. The US Congress, Washington, DC

Jena AB, Philipson TJ (2008) Cost-effectiveness analysis and innovation. J Health Econ 27:1224–1236

Mas-Colell A, Whinston M, Green J (1995) Microeconomic theory. Oxford University Press, New York

Pekarsky BAK (2012) Trust, constraints and the counterfactual: reframing the political economy of new drug price. Dissertation, University of Adelaide http://digital.library.adelaide.edu.au/dspace/handle/2440/79171. Accessed 25 Dec 2013

Reinhardt U (2007) The pharmaceutical sector in health care. In: Sloan F, Hsieh C-R (eds) Pharmaceutical innovation: incentives, competition, and cost-benefit analysis in international perspective. Cambridge University Press, New York

Santerre RE, Vernon JA (2006) Assessing consumer gains from a drug price control policy in the United States. South Econ J 73(1):233–245

Chapter 11
Conclusion

Abstract The concluding chapter presents the guide for regulators to playing and winning the new drug reimbursement game. The results from the previous chapters are summarised as four rules and four tools in this guide. Some of the counterintuitive results from applying these rules are discussed, including the result that if the new drug has additional benefits beyond health gains, that this could lead to a reduced rather that increased threshold. Likely criticisms of these rules by clinicians, social decision makers and some health economists are discussed. The regulator should not respond to these criticisms by increasing the threshold for "special cases". Instead she should present information about the opportunity cost of the strategy to reimburse at a premium above the health shadow price to decision makers. This response goes some way in addressing the failure of the market and institutions to invest in the development of evidence of unpatented interventions. The possibility that the factor that is common to such criticism is that stakeholders value novelty per se and are willing to trade-off population health benefits to gain novelty is introduced.

11.1 The First Problem

The Reimburser looks at her original brief.

- The Minister for Health and the Minister for International Trade ask the Reimburser her opinion on whether applying a decision threshold price per effect for new drugs that is lower than the FPP will lead the population's health to be worse off in the longer run.

Her answer is that if the decision threshold is enforced at an IPER below the FPP, it is likely to lead to improved health for the population in both the short- and long-term, compared with FPP, provided that the threshold is β_c. Also, lowering the price below the FPP is certain to reduce the profits to Pharma, and there is a significant incentive for Pharma to protect these rents.

Then she presents the Ministers with her reframed critical research question.

© Springer International Publishing Switzerland 2015
B.A.K. Pekarsky, *The New Drug Reimbursement Game*,
DOI 10.1007/978-3-319-08903-4_11

• How should a rational Institution respond to the following threat by Pharma? If a purchase price for a new drug is below a FPP, this will lead to:

  – Suboptimal incentives for R&D;
  – Less new drugs in the future; and
  – A future population whose health will be worse that it would otherwise be.

The Reimburser is confident that, if we assume there is no relationship between price and future innovation, β_c is the reimbursement decision threshold that will maximise the health of the population from current and future budgets. β_c achieves this because it:

• Characterises reimbursement as comprising both adoption and displacement and can therefore accommodate inefficiency arising from either or both of these actions, not just resulting from adoption as is the case with conventional CEA and
• Accommodates:

  – Competition in the market for both R&D and current health inputs (as n decreases so does β_c);
  – Inefficiency in displacement ($d < m$);
  – The fixed or constrained budget (there is foregone benefit); and
  – Allocative inefficiency ($m - n > 0$) and technical inefficiency ($m - \mu > 0$).

Furthermore, the use of β_c addresses the market's failure to develop evidence of: (1) unpatented or unpatentable services; or (2) services that will be displaced if evidence of their ICER or IPER is developed (because they are cost ineffective). The use of β_c achieves this by placing an economic (decision) value on the following:

• Of current services (in contraction), m;
• The most cost-effective of current services (in expansion), n;
• The most cost-effective investment strategy μ; and
• The ICER or IPER of services that are displaced, d.

The Reimburser is also confident to state that the evidence of a positive relationship between price and future innovation is not sufficient to establish a case for pricing at the FPP. Furthermore, she has learnt to ask for the derivation of an FPP when firms claim it is the price that will maximise the population's health.

The Reimburser is not willing to say: "There is no situation in which a drug should be reimbursed at a price higher than β_c, in order to account for the relationship between price and innovation." Only two specific reasons why the Reimburser should pay the FPP or a premium were assessed by the Health Economic Adviser (Games 2 and 3). There is no doubt that Pharma will continue to generate more win-win reasons for the FPP. Pharma is behaving exactly as we would expect a large industry protecting its economic rent to behave. However, the Reimburser now has two tools to help her assess any argument put forward by Pharma. The first tool is to analyse the problem as a GTM and not a DTM.

The second tool is a range of parameters that are relevant to assessing the question of pricing higher than β_c including: the IMER of current and future drugs; ΔE^P of the future drug; and the uncertainty surrounding these estimates. She is, however, quietly confident that there is no case that Pharma can present that would result in a premium above β_c. Her confidence has two sources. First, there is significant uncertainty in the characteristics of a future drug, even if it is already in phase 3 clinical trials. Second, the fact that the Institution is more risk-averse than the Capital Market means that Pharma will always prefer the Capital Market option if the Institution seeks a return on its investment in R&D via higher prices that compensates for the associated risk.

Finally, the Reimburser is keen to apply β_c as the new drug decision threshold as soon as possible so that she can redress:

- The long-term failure of the Institution to correct for the failure of the market to provide incentives for the development on unpatented or unpatentable technologies; and
- The additional distortions introduced by generating incentives for firms to price drugs over the economic value of the clinical innovation at the maxWTP.

She is reminded of Arrow (1963):

The social adjustment towards optimality thus puts obstacles in its own path. (p. 947)

11.2   It's About the Journey

The Reimburser notes the other original concepts introduced during her "Adventures in Pharma-land" and realises that to arrive at the simple result of β_c as the maximum acceptable IPER regardless of the relationship between price today and innovation, many smaller simple problems needed to be solved.

With hindsight, she and the Health Economic Adviser realise that seven references were critical to the development of PEA and the health shadow price.

1. Danzig (1963) identifies the competitive nature of an input market, even though a producer of a specific input is a monopolist. The idea that the firm must be paid the maxWTP (appropriate the entire consumer surplus without reference to competition) in order to generate appropriate incentives for R&D neglects this aspect of the economics of the competitive market.
2. McKean (1972) explains, in words, a number of options for calculating a shadow price, and what these options mean.
3. Comanor (1986) clarifies that the political economy of new drugs is dynamic and defines the research agenda, in terms of both inclusion and exclusion criteria.

4. Mishan (1982) critiques Williams "social decision making approach" as an alternative to welfare economic criteria and is a reminder that health economic evaluation could have developed along different paths (the counterfactual).[1]
5. Birch and Gafni (1993) reminds the health economics profession of the centrality of the concept of opportunity cost in the application of economic evaluation to decision making. Ignore it at patients' peril.
6. Mishan and Quah (2007) explains the difference between the shadow price of the budget constraint and the shadow price in CBA.
7. Buchanan (2008) reminds economists of the difference between the operational definition of the counterfactual (alternative strategies available to the decision maker) and the economic concept (the best alternative end state, even if the strategy to achieve this is not directly available to the decision maker).[2]

The smaller problems solved on this journey relate to both pharma-economics and pharmaco-economics.

The issues addressed in relation to pharma-economics follow.

- The recognition that the claim by Pharma that the population will be worse off if prices are lowered is a Threat, with a significant payoff to Pharma if successful. This Threat may or not be supported by the evidence.
- The conventional PEND, and the associated method of calculating rate of return on investment in higher prices excludes the possibility that more drugs in the future will lead to worse health than would otherwise be possible.
- It is possible to have a very high and positive estimate of the conventional rate of rate of return on consumer investment but for this to result in lower health for the population in the future.
- Reframing the political economy of new drugs to include the possibility that more additional drugs will reduce the population's health compared with what would otherwise be the case.

The issues addressed in relation to pharmaco-economics follow.

- The strategy of reimbursement has two actions: adoption and displacement.
- The endogeneity of the price of new drug; it is the result of negotiation, regulation and bargaining power, not the result of an RCT, a systematic review of the literature nor the adjustment of a charge to become a cost. Prices are not constants.

---

[1] "Analyst A" (misrepresenting Mishan) would have been calculating the shadow price of inputs rather than the maxWTP. "Analyst B" could benefit from reading Pekarsky (2012, Appendix 10). "Analyst C" (representing Williams) should not have been excused for ignoring the market's failure to provide evidence of the cost and consequences of unpatented and unpatentable programs. [See Drummond et al. (2005) p. 18 for details of these Analysts]

[2] Some health economists might argue that this is "first best economics gone mad". However, the ongoing neglect of the failure of the market to generate incentives for evidence relating to unpatented or unpatentable programs while generating (inflated) incentives to firms to provide evidence of patented technologies is a consequence of the neglect of the first best world.

The IPER, IMER, and IπER, which were developed to facilitate the math, highlight different sources of innovation (including manufacturing innovation) and the appropriation of economic rent from previous innovative NMEs by subsequent NMEs.

- The distinction between types of budgets: fixed, constrained, unconstrained and no budget.
- The use of game theory to engage with Pharma's rent-seeking (lobbying).
- The idea of a health shadow price that accommodates allocative or technical inefficiency as competition in the institution's market for health inputs.
- PEA, which compares the effect of the strategy of reimbursement on the population with the best alternative strategy, giving a value to the evidence of the counterfactual.

The Reimburser also acknowledges that there are many opportunities for further research. For example, expected value of information methods such as those described in Drummond et al. (2005) and by Eckermann and Willan (2007) could be used to identify and quantify the value of reducing the uncertainty around β_c. Conventional expected value of information methods could be adapted to accommodate endogeneity of the new drug price, which is assumed to be exogenous in current models. But is all this enough to ensure that β_c will be adopted as the threshold price?

11.3 The Next Problem

The Reimburser is surprised when a chorus of criticism of β_c as the decision threshold of choice emanates from, not Pharma and pharma-economists, but the health economic community. She identifies nine arguments against using β_c and for using either k or d. She is also provided with a book chapter by a US health economist that suggests a theoretical approach to incorporating the cost of R&D in a CEA (Pauly 2007). Each of these arguments are addressed in the following sections.

11.3.1 Benefits Beyond QALYs

The first criticism is that β_c assumes that there is no benefit from a new drug other than the incremental QALYs. There are many cases when a new drug has additional benefits beyond health, for example, it could also improve productivity. Alternatively, the new drug could address "equity" in situations where patients with end-stage cancer have no other treatment options. Finally, characteristics of patients such as disease severity could also be seen to have a value independent of capacity to benefit in terms of health effects.

The Reimburser is so confident in the answer to this question that she does not even ask her Health Economist Adviser. She refers to Chap. 6 and shows that if the objective of the reimbursement process is changed to, for example, "QALY plus other thing", so should the set of alternative strategies from which the best alternative strategy is selected. If the impact of the drug on factors such as productivity and equity are measurable and valued, then any means of achieving the same outcomes should be assessed. In fact, if the additional non-health benefits of the new drug are also valued, then it is possible that the most cost-effective alternative strategy results in a shadow price lower than β_c, a "health+" shadow price; a counterintuitive but plausible result. [See Pekarsky (2012, Appendix 10) for an example of this situation.]

11.3.2   But No One Will Implement the Best Alternative Strategy

The second criticism is: what if β_c is applied, the new drug is rejected because $f > \beta_c$, but then the best alternative strategy is not adopted? The Reimburser is confused. What does this mean? Is this concern simply a justification for the decision to reimburse the new drug at a higher threshold? This justification is underpinned by the following or similar logic.

- If we reject the drug at the offer IPER because $f > \beta_c$ even though $d > f$, no one will actually perform the reallocation to the best alternative strategy. Therefore, we might as well just reimburse at f because at least the population's health will increase.

In this case the appropriate response is to explicate and solve the following paradox:

- Why would an Institution not adopt an alternative more effective strategy, but be willing to reimburse the new drug instead, even if this action foregoes the more cost-effective opportunity?

Perhaps the costs of reducing allocative efficiency are too high? If there are costs to improving allocative efficiency, then these should be incorporated into the estimate of the β_c by redefining the set of alternative strategies. However, in this case the costs of the uptake of significant new drugs should also be included in the IPER, for example, the ongoing costs of prescriber education programs. Any reason that an Institution can give to not adopt the more effective strategy should be analysed and, where appropriate, accommodated in the estimate of β_c. What if all of the possible explanations are exhausted and a reluctance to implement the best alternative strategy remains? Then it is a question of "finding the market or institutional failure", that is, working out why the Institution will not implement the better strategy.

11.3.3   Decision Makers Need to Understand the Health Shadow Price

The third criticism is: What if the Social Decision Maker[3] cannot understand why he should use β_c rather than the maxWTP? This criticism is slightly harder to address. An intuitive explanation for using β_c is quite simple: this is the lowest ICER at which the health budget holder could use the funds required to finance the incremental cost of the new drug to purchase QALYs from some other source. So why might the Social Decision Maker not understand this definition?

It could be because the Social Decision Maker does not understand the idea or consequence of a budget constraint. It could be because he has conflated the idea of displacement and opportunity cost. It could be that he is convinced of the price-innovation relationship as evidence of the need to price at high thresholds. Any of these issues could be resolved by a bit of education.

However, the preference for the maxWTP as the threshold could be a consequence of a Social Decision Maker being *unwilling to accept* rather than *unable to understand* the difference between a shadow price and a maxWTP (Chap. 5). This scenario introduces another possibility:

- The Social Decision Maker seeks to maximise the number of new technologies funded;
- He works within the constraint of the lay concept of economic accountability (value for money); and hence
- The preference for the maxWTP rather than the shadow price is a preference for the maximum possible threshold that is also accountable.

That is, the maxWTP threshold maximises the number of new drugs funded, with the minimum of delay, while meeting the constraint of "value for money", as understood in the lay sense.

One possible response to this situation is to provide the Social Decision Maker with evidence of the health effects lost for patients whose services are displaced (d) or forgone yet to be expanded (n). Then the net economic loss of reimbursement at thresholds above β_c can be expressed as a trade-off between health gains for the target patients and forgone benefit to other patients and, if necessary, the Social Decision Maker's preference for "new technology" can be derived. The forgone benefit to these patients could be documented in as rich detail as the benefits of reimbursement to target patients for the new drug. The Social Decision Maker might not understand the economics behind this comparison. However, improving the comparability of the depth and breadth of evidence of the potential and forgone

---

[3] For a discussion of this character, see the Glossary of Characters. This is the Social Decision maker that Analyst C provides information to [See Drummond et al. (2005) p. 18].

benefits of the decision of reimbursement should go some way in personalising the foregone benefit.[4]

If the Social Decision Maker chooses to reimburse the new drug, even if there is an economic loss, then at least the decision can be framed as one that reveals a preference for the method of production (new things) rather than a preference for health benefits to patients.

11.3.4   Social Decision Makers Do Not Understand Opportunity Cost

Clinicians appear to find the concept of opportunity cost difficult to understand and hence this lack of understanding seems to become a justification for not using it to guide decisions. Alternatively social decision makers could argue that opportunity cost is "not a concrete concept".

As discussed in Chap. 4, opportunity cost in the economic sense is analogous to the decision by health technology assessment groups to use the most effective current treatment for the specified clinical context as the comparator against which a new drug is compared in order to determine its clinically innovative value. The benefit of the new drug is determined by comparing it to the best alternative strategy—the benefit that must be foregone to the patient in order for it to obtain the benefits of the new drug; the opportunity cost of using the drug for that patient.

Pekarsky (2012, Appendix 11) includes a presentation that the Health Economist used to explain to the Reimburser (and other pharmaco-economists and health economists) the relationship between opportunity cost in a clinical and economic context and why the economic value of a new drug can only be calculated with reference to the loss from the best alternative strategy.

11.3.5   Reimbursement of the New Drug and Reallocation Are Not Mutually Exclusive Strategies

"The funder could both reimburse the new drug and reallocate resources; they are not mutually exclusive strategies in the same way that choosing to build a new road through a city using either route A or Route B are," said the Operations Research expert.

---

[4] Towse (2010, p 316) describes this problem as comparing the benefits to a "known" group of patients with the potential loss to an unknown group of patients whose health benefits are foregone. He describes the choice of decision threshold as being a choice between a choice between a "known group of patients against the unknown" and the choice of valuing the unknown patients' foregone benefits above those of the known patients' benefits as "pessimistic".

This is true; the budget holder could fund reimbursement and perform reallocation. However, this does not mean that the strategy of improving efficiency (reallocation or investing in improved practice) is not the strategy against which reimbursement should be compared to determine whether the strategy of reimbursement has a net economic cost or benefit. Without a reference strategy, the question of whether there is an economic benefit to the strategy of reimbursement cannot be answered.

But is choosing a reference strategy a complex problem? It is not complex when we are choosing between Routes A and B for a motorway that will maximise the number of people who can be transported in peak hour, given a budget. Nor is it complex when we are choosing between Drugs A and B in order to maximise the health benefit for the patient given that the patent can only have one course of medications. The complexity occurs when we consider that there may be other actions outside those nominated above that could be more effective at achieving the goals of improved transport at peak hours and improved population health respectively. These strategies include reducing the number of cars or improving respite care, both of which could be currently unfunded. It becomes even more complex when the endogeneity of price and hence strategy cost is considered. If improved efficiency is not considered as a reference strategy, the possibility that a population will benefit if a firm lowers the price of the new drug to be more competitive with other strategies available to the Reimburser. The critical issue is that economics considers the possibility that there is market and/or institutional failure in the process for nominating the nominated strategies from which the best option is selected.

PEA provides a framework that corrects for the reasons why an Institution will continue to adopt a new drug based on evidence of its incremental cost and effect, even though strategies that are preferable to it continue to go unfunded. If instead we say both strategies could both be implemented and hence we should just continue to reimburse, the question of "what is the threshold price" remains unanswered and the probability that the more cost-effective strategies are never funded also remains high. The consequence is that at any point in time in the future the population's health will be less than what it could have been had the reference strategy been recognised and firms either forced to change their price or the reference strategy adopted.

Another way of considering this issue is to invert the well-known story of how to find the shadow price of the budget constraint by starting with an unallocated budget and allocating funds to each project, ranked by decreasing cost-effectiveness (See Sect. 8.9.3.1) until the budget is exhausted. This problem defines the optimum set of rules by which an unallocated budget can be allocated so as to maximise the health benefits possible. In this case we start with a fully allocated budget that is allocatively inefficient. We recognise that an institution could potentially implement both the strategy of reimbursement of the new drug and the strategy of improving allocative inefficiency; these strategies are not functionally mutually exclusive in the way that choosing between the Routes A and B to build a motorway are.

The problem is to select from two mutually exclusive sets of rules that can be used to address each successive reimbursement decision.

The first set of rules is to adopt the health shadow price and apply this as a threshold price for the health effects from a new drug; adopt PEA. The second set of rules is to continue to implement both of these strategies (reimbursement and improved efficiency), and to repeat this each time a new drug is considered for reimbursement. Which of these two rules will be certain to have the higher health benefits at each point in time? Which of these two rules provides a clear signal to the firm as to the value ion exchange of a health effect? How is the threshold price selected in the second set of rules? Now take into account the complexities such as, under reimbursement institution rules, the new drug cannot be displaced to finance a future new unrelated drug, only unpatented programs can be displaced.

It is true that the two strategies of reimbursement and improving efficiency are not functionally mutually exclusive, however, in order to maximise the health of a population from a given budget over successive reimbursement decisions, it is necessary to minimise the economic cost of each decision. In order to use the first set of rules, a reference strategy is necessary in order to estimate economic loss and to send a price signal to the firm. The only reference strategy that is grounded in economic theory is the strategy with the largest net effect on the population, the strategy to improve efficiency.

11.3.6 The Decision Threshold Should Not Be Revealed to the Industry

The next criticism is that the decision threshold should not be revealed to the firm and that instead the institution should keep it as private information and use this private information to bargain a price below the threshold. At first glance this appears to address the problem of firms pricing at the maximum price (their best response to a revealed maximum) and seems to introduce the possibility that the price will be lower that would otherwise be the case. There are two reasons why the simple bilateral bargaining model such as wage bargaining model will not lead to the result of maximising population's health by increasing the proportion of decisions that have their price below the shadow price.

First, the objective of this exercise of using the health shadow price is to provide a signal to manufacturers and other advocates, agents and owners of inputs of the cheapest way that an incremental health effect can be obtained. It is about addressing the markets' failure to supply such a price and to develop evidence of the effectiveness of unpatentable and unpatented technologies.

Furthermore, the critical problem faced by reimbursing authorities is not how far they bargain below the decision threshold, but how to counteract the pressure to price above any price that they nominate as a maximum price. This characteristic of the PEND is why the decision to impose a decision threshold is characterised as price control: the argument from Pharma is to not go below the firms' preferred price, which is higher than the institutions preferred price, whatever that institution's price is. This is why the US pharma-economists characterise a free market in pharmaceuticals as a unilateral rather than a bilateral monopoly where only firms have market power [See Pekarsky (2012, Appendix 7)].

Therefore, the decision threshold that is the health shadow price should not only be in the public domain, empirical evidence to support its value should be valued at least as much as the evidence of the ICER of a new drug and the social value of investing in this evidence should be recognised.

11.3.7 The Games Only Apply to the Australian Setting

"This story is a thinly disguised narrative of the Australian experience over the 20 years since 1991 since economic evaluation first started to be used for new drug. It has limited relevance to the rest of the OECD" said the European health economist.

Some characteristics of the games and stories are strongly reflective of the Australian experience; this is true. However characteristics of the PEND, the structure of the games and the narrative are common to all countries that use economic evaluation to inform the decisions about new drugs. Games can be uniquely specified using the different reimbursement rules in each country and then solved for the different strategies adopted by Pharma. Furthermore, the novel aspects of the solution (the use of game theory, the IMER, IPER and IπER to specify a firm production function and the health shadow price) provide the economic tools with which a country specific game constructed. These tools represent a new way to engage in the political economy of new drug price. These games and the methods are in the public domain; they have value if they are adapted and used by institutions.

11.3.8 What About the Political Cost of Reallocation?

"But there is a political cost to reallocating, otherwise we would already adopted this strategy" said the employee of a major European public health authority. This is partly true; political costs of actions do mean that the strategy that maximises the health of the population will not necessarily be implemented.

First, political cost is only one reason that this reallocation, while population health improving, has not yet occurred. A second reason is the market's and institution's failure to generate the necessary evidence and to provide an institution path by which strategies that are cost-effective can be implemented and the resultant decision protected from displacement. Hence, the use of the health shadow price corrects for this failure of market and institutions to provide evidence.

Second, even if this alternative strategy is identified and it is considered too politically costly to implement it and the drug is reimbursed instead, there is an opportunity to translate this political cost to a health cost. Under PEA and the health shadow price, institutions are presented with as much information about the health gain to the patients who could benefit from reallocation (and those who will lose) as they are of the information about the services that will be displaced and the health benefits of the new drug. Hence, the market's and institutions failure to reveal the health cost of not undertaking a reallocation can be addressed at least partly and this cost put into the public domain and compared to the benefits of reimbursement of the new drug.

Third, it would be useful for the political cost to be converted to units such as health gains foregone in order to compare it to the economic cost of not implementing the strategy of improved efficiency. The economic cost of reimbursing but not improving efficiency is clear—it is a loss in population health gains compared to what would otherwise occur. It is unclear how the politicians compare the political cost to the economic cost or improving efficiency. Do politicians have a sense of the economic cost or does it have no value in their decision making?

And finally, if this alternative strategy is identified and it is politically costly to implement, that does not necessarily mean that the new drug should be reimbursed. Are there other strategies that are preferable to reimbursement that are less politically costly? Alternatively is the problem that Institutions are so convinced by the conventional political economy of new drugs that they are unwilling to challenge this conventional wisdom lest they make significant losses in areas such as increased barriers to agricultural exports.

11.3.9 The Costs of R&D Can Be Incorporated into a CEA

The next criticism is that the costs of R&D should be incorporated into the CEA to determine the price that optimises the incentives for innovation (Pauly 2007). Pauly's method incorporates factors that determine extent and distribution of R&D that are not considered in this book, such as countries with different regulatory structures and the incentive to invest in one country rather than another. However, it is important to note that his discussion does not refer to the competition from other sources of inputs or innovation. Nor does Pauly refer to the potential for firms to make strategic use of private information about the costs of R&D and the marginal costs of production of drugs. He assumes this information will be supplied—placed in the public domain—even though this could be to the firm's disadvantage. He also assumes firms will not be strategic in exactly which information they put in the public domain, that is, they will be honest and fully reveal the true costs of R&D.

11.3.10 There Is No Evidence of n, d, m, and μ

Most significantly, it could be argued that there are no estimates of the parameters: n, d, m, and μ.

The Reimburser notes that some pharma-economists have accepted the argument that the FPP is the price that will optimise future innovation without requiring evidence of the value of that future innovation (ΔE of the future drug) or the maths used to derive this FPP.

She offers five starting points for health economists who wish to make headway into an otherwise intractable problem: we can't apply the health shadow price because we do not know its value but we do not know its value unless we provide a value for this evidence.

1. There are two aspects to reducing uncertainty in the estimate of β_c. Uncertainty as to which programmes and technologies correspond to n, d, m, and μ and uncertainty as to the value of the ICER or IPER of each of these programmes.
2. The expected cost of reducing uncertainty in the estimate of these parameters depends upon a number of factors, including the currently preferred threshold. If the currently preferred threshold is k then estimates of all three parameters need to be obtained. If the current preferred estimate is d and this is accompanied by a strategy to reduce the inefficiency of displacement (identification of m), then the only additional parameter that needs to be estimated is n.
3. The value of reducing uncertainty also depends upon the current choice of threshold; the greater the economic loss associated with the prevailing threshold, the greater the value of evidence β_c, the greater the incentive to generate evidence. The economic loss (health) of each decision to reimburse a new drug of additional cost ΔC^P, using the current threshold CEA_i where $i > \beta_c$ and the Firm prices at i, is given by:

$$\Delta C^P (i - \beta_c).$$

In the case of CEA_d which is accompanied by a strategy of disinvestment,[5] the value of reducing uncertainty in the value of β_c increases and the cost of reducing this uncertainty decreases over time. The logic follows.

(a) Assume that k provides an upper limit to the choice of threshold;
(b) As the efficiency of displacement increases, d approaches m;
(c) Hence the economic loss of using the preferred threshold, approaches the economic loss associated with k;

---

[5] There is now a sizeable body of literature looking at the practicalities and merits of disinvestment strategies. A number of the studies associated with NICE also raise the relationship with the choice of threshold (Culyer et al. 2007; Elshaug et al. 2007; Pearson and Littlejohns 2007; Walker et al. 2007).

(d) However, as more reliable estimates of d and m become available, then the incremental cost of evidence of β_c reduces; the only additional parameter that needs to be estimated is n.

4. There is no requirement to identify the shadow price of the budget constraint (in expansion) λ_e^B in order to make an estimate of β_c. The analogous parameter in PEA is n, the most cost-effective programme in expansion or most cost-effective unfunded programme or technology; it is a concrete rather than abstract concept.

5. A first cut set of parameter estimates could be obtained relatively easily. Vernon et al. (2010) required an estimate of the least cost-effective of existing programmes to estimate the full value threshold. The authors' choice of the ICER of dialysis is probably a reasonable starting point in most health systems for the estimate of m. The weighted average ICER of programmes that were contracted or not implemented in the last round of health budget cuts is d. Then the value of n could be the first programme that could be expanded or implemented and has an ICER $> (d - m)$. This will ensure that the first approximation of β_c is above zero.[6]

11.4 Postscript

For more than 20 years, the Reimburser had thought that in order to win the best deal for her population it was simply necessary to:

- Ensure that the best evidence of incremental cost and incremental effect was made available to the Institution;
- Develop and present this information in a way that is consistent with a protocol that is responsive to evolving methods;
- Evaluate this information for quality and accuracy; and
- Compare the resultant ICER to a decision threshold and if it is above this threshold, the beyond QALY benefits and opportunities to decrease price are negotiated.

She now recognises that the price that is the input into this cost-effectiveness analysis is set strategically. She also recognises that not all information that appears to be based in evidence is what it appears to be, particularly claims about information such as the return to higher prices. She sets herself a challenge: summarise PEA as a strategy and a set of tools.

---

[6] The Reimburser has grown to be quite tolerant of hard-core economics. However, if $\beta_C < 0$ because the existing budget has significant allocative inefficiency ... well, she can see the headlines now—"Companies asked to pay the government if drugs are innovative". She understands that this will not necessarily be the effect of a threshold below zero, and firms could still make an economic profit on these drug sales (see Chaps. 8, 9 and 10). But why let economic sense stand in the way of a good headline? Such is the political economy of new drugs.

First, she synthesises the lessons as a four part strategy that should be followed to play and win the new drug reimbursement game.

A Strategy with Four Rules

1. Drug pricing is a game and the regulators make and enforce the rules.
2. Recognise that resources are constrained. If a new drug is reimbursed at an additional financial cost to the health budget, something, somewhere, will need to be displaced to finance it. It is likely that no health budget can be expanded to accommodate all purchases that are considered "value for money" in the lay sense of the term.
3. Recognise that firms will act strategically. A rational firm will employ strategies to maximise their economic rent and the higher the potential rent the more a firm will invest into protecting or attracting that rent.
4. Never accept a price above the health shadow price without a contract with the firm that specifies the investment and return to the health budget.

Then she lists the four tools that are available to the health economist that acts to advise a regulator.

Tools

1. A decision threshold that captures existing technical and allocative inefficiency and suboptimal displacement; the health shadow price, β_c.
2. A notation for the ICER of a new drug—the IPER—that captures the endogeneity of the price of the drug to the pricing process and the economic context.
3. Two metrics that allow that allow the firm's cost and profit function for a new drug to be specified in incremental health effect of the new drug (the same units as the production function for the health budget): the IMER and the IπER.
4. Three examples of games that can be adapted to accommodate and assess any Threat claimed by a firm as part of a drug pricing process as the justification for maintaining a price above the decision threshold—and the contract that recognises the public's investment and return as a general solution to any version of this game.

References

Buchanan J (2008) Opportunity cost. In: Durlauf S, Blume L (eds) The New Palgrave dictionary of economics online, 2nd edn. Palgrave Macmillian, Basingstoke

Birch S, Gafni A (1993b) Changing the problem to fit the solution: Johannesson and Weinstein's (mis) application of economics to real-world problems. J Health Econ 12(4):469–476

Comanor WS (1986) The political economy of the pharmaceutical industry. J Econ Lit 24 (3):1178–1217

Culyer A, McCabe C, Briggs A, Claxton K, Buxton M, Akehurst R, Sculpher M, Brazier J (2007) Searching for a threshold, not setting one: the role of the National Institute for Health and Clinical Excellence. J Health Serv Res Policy 12(1):56–58. doi:10.1258/135581907779497567

Danzig G (1963) Linear programming and extensions. Reports, vol R-366_PR. RAND Corporation, Santa Monica, CA

Drummond MF, Sculpher MJ, Torrance GW, O'Brien BJ, Stoddart GL (2005) Methods for the economic evaluation of health care programmes, 3rd edn. Oxford University Press, Oxford

Eckermann S, Willan A (2007) Expected value of information and decision making in HTA. Health Econ 16(2):195–209

Elshaug A, Hiller J, Tunis S, Moss J (2007) Challenges in Australian policy processes for disinvestment from existing, ineffective health care practices. Aust New Zealand Health Policy 4(23)

McKean RN (1972) The use of shadow prices. In: Layard R (ed) Cost benefit analysis. Penguin, Harmondsworth, pp 119–139

Mishan E (1982) The new controversy about the rationale of economic evaluation. J Econ Issues XVI(1):29–47

Mishan E, Quah E (2007) Cost-benefit analysis, 5th edn. Routledge, Abingdon

Pauly M (2007) Measures of costs and benefits for drugs in cost-effectiveness research. In: Sloan F, Hsieh C-R (eds) Pharmaceutical innovation: incentives, competition, and cost-benefit analysis in international perspective. Cambridge University Press, New York, pp 199–214

Pearson S, Littlejohns P (2007) Reallocating resources: how should the National Institute for Health and Clinical Excellence guide disinvestment efforts in the National Health Service? J Health Serv Res Policy 12(3):160–165. doi:10.1258/135581907781542987

Pekarsky BAK (2012) Trust, constraints and the counterfactual: reframing the political economy of new drug price. Dissertation, University of Adelaide http://digital.library.adelaide.edu.au/dspace/handle/2440/79171. Accessed 25 Dec 2013

Towse A (2010) Value based pricing, research and development, and patient access schemes. Will the United Kingdom get it right or wrong? Br J Clin Pharmacol 70(3):360–366. doi:10.1111/j.1365-2125.2010.03740.x

Vernon JA, Golec JH, Stevens JS (2010) Comparative effectiveness regulations and pharmaceutical innovation. Pharmacoeconomics 28(10):877–887

Walker S, Palmer S, Sculpher M (2007) The role of NICE technology appraisal in NHS rationing. Br Med Bull 81–82:51–64. doi:10.1093/bmb/ldm007

Glossary of Characters

Firm	The capitalised "Firm" refers to a player in a Game. It is introduced in Game 1, Chap. 8 and it features in Games 2 and 3 in Chaps. 9 and 10 respectively. It is capitalised, as is the convention in Game theory models. It has specific production functions and markets.
firm	A firm with a small "f" is a pharmaceutical firm with no specific cost function who participates in the reimbursement process, invests in R&D and lobbies for higher prices. Its objective function is profit maximisation.
Institution	The capitalised "Institution" refers to a specific institution that is a player in a Game. In these Games the Institution needs to consider how to respond to a threat from Pharma or a specific Firm. It has specific rules it must play by.
institution	And institution with a small "i" is the collective term for the regulators involved in decisions about new drugs. The institutions of interest in this book are those that work in countries that use cost-effectiveness analysis to make decisions about the reimbursement of new drugs, have universal health care schemes and constrained budgets.
Reimburser	The Reimburser is the key character in this book. She is neither an economist nor a clinician. She is bureaucrat who works with a clear objective function: to maximise the health gains possible from this and future budgets.
Health Economic Adviser	The Health Economic Adviser is the second character in this book. His task is to take the problems presented to him by the Reimburser and apply economic theory to solve them.
Pharma	Pharma is the name given to the pharmaceutical industry, particularly those firms that invests in R&D.

Displacer   The Displacer's job description is to "find savings" in order
                          to allow for the additional costs of programs such as the drug
                          budget to be financed. He may or may not be able to find the
                          least cost-effective of existing programs and if he does he
                          cannot always displace them. In most cases, he cannot
                          displace patented health technologies.

Social decision   Drummond et al. (2005, p 18) refer to three types of
maker   Analysts: A, B and C. Analyst C takes the position that the
                          role of the economic analyst is to provide information on a
                          "wide range of costs and consequences and present them in a
                          way that helps health care decision makers form a better
                          judgement".
                               The Social Decision Maker referred to in this book is the
                          person in receipt of this information. He is not an economist.
                          He is probably a clinician. He may have a preference for
                          particular method of production, specifically, he may prefer
                          to use a new drug rather than an existing drug, even if it is no
                          more effective, because he values "newness".

Glossary of Phrases

Universal health care	The term universal health care is used to distinguish between the health care schemes in counties such as the US and other developed countries such as Canada, Australia, New Zealand, England, Scotland, Denmark, Sweden, Finland, Norway and the Netherlands. The latter counties have not achieved equitable access to a minimum level of care for all patients and significant disparities in utilisation and health outcomes remain. In Australia, the gap in access to health care for Indigenous Australian compared to non-Indigenous Australians contributes to the significant gap in life expectancy at birth for males.
New drug price	New drug price refers to the phenomena of new drug price as the focus of heated debate. It refers to all new drugs, not a specific new drug.
Political economy of new drugs	The political economy of new drugs (PEND) is the economic expression of the heated debate about how the surplus associated with a new drug's innovation should be allocated across consumers, institutional purchasers and firms via price mechanisms.
Policy narrative	The policy narrative is the story that surrounds the development and implementation of a policy, such as how to regulate the price of new drugs. It could be a simple cause and effect narrative and may or may not make reference to evidence.
Evidence based policy narrative	The evidence based narrative is a term I use to describe a policy narrative that is populated by multiple references to empirical evidence but not

© Springer International Publishing Switzerland 2015
B.A.K. Pekarsky, *The New Drug Reimbursement Game*,
DOI 10.1007/978-3-319-08903-4

	evidence that justifies the actual policy choice. For example, reference to the burden of disease associated with a condition to justify a policy to screen for a condition, with no reference to the evidence of the effectiveness of that program in reducing that burden of disease.
New drug, new NME	The new drug or new NME has recently been approved for prescribing by the FDA or an equivalent national agency and now prices are being negotiated. Evidence of incremental cost and effect are available.
Future drug, future NME	The future drug is one that has not yet completed phase 3 trials or the molecule has not even been discovered. Evidence of incremental cost and effect is not available.
Future population's health	One of the objectives of the conventional political economy of new drugs is to identify the health of a future population with or without additional future drugs. Of course it is by and large today's population, just older, and with different medical technologies.
Present value of population's future health	The present value of the population's future health is the PV of expected life time health of a population in the future—not just the health in 1 year.
Net present value population's health	This is the previous concept less the loss in health effects today as a consequence of higher prices today and hence less health today.

Glossary of Prices and Costs in Price-Effectiveness Analysis

FPP	The firm's preferred price is the price that the firm offers a new drug at and also a price that the firm justifies as the price that should be used.
PPP	The purchaser's preferred price is the price that a purchaser believes maximises the objectives, whatever these are. The purchaser might be making a "mistake"
IPER, f	The incremental price-effectiveness ratio is arithmetically identical to the ICER but price is recognised as endogenous and a function of the choice of the decision threshold rather than as exogenous.
IMER	The incremental cost to the firm of producing the incremental health effect compared to the previous drug.
IπER	The incremental economic rent to the firm on the incremental health effect.

© Springer International Publishing Switzerland 2015
B.A.K. Pekarsky, *The New Drug Reimbursement Game*,
DOI 10.1007/978-3-319-08903-4

Glossary of Notation and Parameters

β_c The health shadow price: the aICER of the most cost-effective strategy to increase the population's health where this strategy will typically include a combination of financing and expenditure. It is a function of the economic context, c, which includes the amount of resources that need to be displaced in order to finance a new drug, the prevailing prices of inputs and the existing degree of inefficiency in the health budget.

N The aICER of the most cost-effective program or technology in expansion or adoption.

M The aICER of the most cost-effective program or technology in contraction or disinvestment.

D The aICER of the program or technology that is displaced to finance the additional costs of the new drug.

R The conventionally measured rate of return on new drugs.

C The IMER in algebraic form. Can vary across drugs.

ΔL^P The additional life years experienced by patients from a new drug or new drugs.

$\mathcal{R}$ The investment in R&D by the firm.

E One alternative expression of return on R&D, incorporating the budget constraint.

F The algebraic expression of the IPER at which the firm offers a new drug.

ω The share of additional economic rent from higher prices that is allocated to new drug R&D.

H The investment by public sector research groups in pharmaceutical R&D.

λ The conventional shadow price of the budget constraint defined by relaxing the budget constraint by one unit.

ΔC^P The incremental cost to the health budget of the new drug at the given price.

© Springer International Publishing Switzerland 2015
B.A.K. Pekarsky, *The New Drug Reimbursement Game*,
DOI 10.1007/978-3-319-08903-4

ΔE	The net increase in the health of the population due to any cause or combination of causes
	The following are all net changes in health to a specific group of patients as a consequence of a specific action or strategy (two actions)
ΔE^A	(A) reallocation from least to most cost-effective of existing programs.
ΔE^D	(D) displacing the program that
ΔE^M	(M) expanding or contracting the least cost-effective program.
ΔE^N	(N) expanding or contracting the most cost-effective program
ΔE^P	(P) from the adoption of a new drug
ΔE^R	(R) from the strategy of reimbursement (the net effect of the new drug and the services displaced to finance it.
ΔE^T	(T) the most cost-effective alternative strategy to reimbursement.
NEBh^R	Net economic benefit of the decision to reimburse, expressed in health units.
EVCI	The economic value of clinical innovation
β_c^α	The health shadow price corresponding to the alternative strategy set which comprises all possible opportunities to reallocate.
β_c^v	As above but corresponding to all investment strategies.
μ	The parameter that defines the increased productivity of a program if there is an investment in improving its technical efficiency.
λ_e^B	The shadow price of the budget constraint (B) defined in expansion (e)
$\lambda_{e|c}^B$	The shadow price of the budget constraint (B) defined in expansion (e), given previous contraction (c).
θ	The interest rate charged by the Capital Market to the Firm, over the period of a loan to finance R&D
κ	A constant that characterises the relationship between clinical innovation of the current drug and the clinical innovation of a future drug.
τ	The interest rate charged by the Capital Market to a zero-risk borrower.
CEAi	Cost-effective analysis applied to inform reimbursement decision, using a threshold of i to correspond to either a NB or an ICER metric
ICERi	The conventional ICER compared to a threshold of i
NBi	The conventional net benefit calculated using i
A	The best alternative strategy to reimbursement that is a reallocation (contraction of least cost-effective to financing of most cost-effective)
R	The strategy of Reimbursement, which comprises adoption and financing. (Not to be confused with $\mathcal{R}$, which is the amount invested into R&D)
T	The best alternative strategy to Reimbursement

Printed in the United States
By Bookmasters